Bringing Up Baby

The First Twelve Months

Ann and Nevin Kishbaugh

Pediatric commentary by Marie Keith, M.D., affiliated with St. Vincent's Hospital in New York

Child Development commentary by Anita Landau Hurtig, Ph.D., of the University of Illinois at Chicago

Bonus Books Inc., Chicago

95   94   93   92   91   5   4   3   2   1

Library of Congress Catalog Card Number: 91-71892

International Standard Book Number: 0-929387-25-2

Bonus Books, Inc.
160 East Illinois Street
Chicago, Illinois 60611

Printed in the United States of America

Bringing Up Baby

With love to the memory of

Ruth Kishbaugh

Our mother, our friend

Contents

Foreword

Bringing Up Baby is about the first twelve months in the life of Adelyn Ruth Kishbaugh, which means it is about growing up and changing. In this book, Addie grows from a tiny, squalling infant to a baby-fat, not-quite toddler. She changes from a dependent, sleeping-most-of-the-time human to a determined, responsive little lady. Addie is just about as normal—and as wonderful—as a baby can be.

But *Bringing Up Baby* is about much more than Addie's first year; it's really about parenting. *Bringing Up Baby* describes how Addie's mother and father, Ann and Nevin, grew and changed during their first year as parents. They share their year with us, a year that is monumental in every new parent's life. Before you meet them and Addie, I'd like to explain how Ann and Nevin met.

In 1981, eight years before Addie was born, I was working as an editor for a small publishing company in Thorofare, New Jersey, and Ann Sandt was my assistant. As the work load increased, management decided we could add an additional assistant. Nevin Kishbaugh applied for the job, and personnel brought him in for an interview.

As I walked to meet Nevin, I scanned his resume, noting grimly that he was a blackjack dealer. Terrific. Personnel seemed to have nothing better to do than waste my time. Feeling frustrated and impatient, I decided I'd talk with this Nevin briefly, just long enough to be polite, and then send him back to Atlantic City to deal cards. I had magazines to get out.

Nevin was seated in a small, straight-backed chair in the middle of our president's office, which happened to be the only space available at that time for the interview. All he needed to complete the "interrogation" scene was a bare bulb swinging over his head. Nevin looked uncomfortable but responded with enthusiasm when I started asking about his qualifications. He had, after all, worked for a newspaper during college. My impatience began to ebb.

I don't remember our conversation, but I do remember my thoughts: "Here's a nice kid with a passion for words and pictures who'd probably work well with Ann Sandt. In fact, (and I felt a swinging bulb go on over *my* head) wouldn't he and Ann make a nice couple?"

To this day, I've no idea why I had that thought at that time. I knew Ann well—she's sweet, smart, conscientious and a pleasure to be around. Here I was mentally matching her up with an unknown blackjack dealer—and at that point she already was matched up with another man.

Of course, I also had my professionalism. Nevin was no less qualified than other candidates I had interviewed, clearly competent and obviously anxious to get started on a new career. We were talking about an entry level position, not the presidency. Besides, his photography skills might come in handy some day.

After Nevin was hired, the three of us worked very hard and the light bulb basically disappeared—except on Monday mornings when everyone talked about their weekends. Ann would tell Nevin, sometimes in detail, what she had done during the weekend with her boyfriend. Nonplussed, Nevin had his own stories. Each Monday morning I'd listen to the chatter and mentally wish Ann's boyfriend away. Then I'd forget about it until the next Monday morning.

Soon we all were promoted. Ann moved up with me and Nevin began to work for another editor. He hated it, began to think more seriously about becoming a professional photographer, and finally left the firm. On the home front, Ann finally ended her relationship with her boyfriend. We were much too busy to talk about it. I forgot about the light bulb.

Then one day, Ann shyly entered my office, closed the door and said, "I have something to tell you." Slight pause. "Nevin and I have been dating." "How nice," I answered, feeling a warm glow as the bulb heated up. "There's more," she added. "We're, well, we're in love." The light bulb was glowing and my tongue was aching as I bit it to keep from exclaiming: "I knew it, I knew it."

This story is as true as Addie is alive and wonderful. Ann and Nevin eventually were married. I struggled with feelings of responsibility for the success or failure of their lives together, but my perspective soon took over. That light bulb was real, very real, but my role was small, less weighty, even, than the long-winded minister who offered endless words of advice at their wedding ceremony. The rest was up to Ann and Nevin. And over the years, with absolutely no help from me or the minister, Ann and Nevin have built a solid relationship of which I stand in awe.

With support from Ann, Nevin did set himself up as a professional photographer. Eventually Ann, too, left publishing and now works as a freelance writer and editor. So together they are a sort of cottage industry—a prolific industry. One day I received a letter to announce that I would soon be a Great Aunt or a Grand Aunt or "whatever you want to call yourself," Ann said.

Meanwhile I'd moved to New York City and was working as the managing editor of *Baby Talk* magazine, the oldest baby magazine in the United States. The publication has a tradition: Each year it follows, month by month, the changes that occur during a baby's first year.

Soon that tradition and the impending birth of Baby Kishbaugh began to meld in my head and another light bulb went on. The timing was perfect and the parents were professionals—a writer and a photographer. I described Ann and Nevin to Susan Strecker, *Baby Talk's* Editor-in-Chief. She agreed to meet with them, liked what she saw and heard, and so *Bringing Up Baby* (not to mention Addie) was born.

I came home late on September 30, 1989, to hear an excited Nevin on my answering machine: "It's a girl, a beautiful girl. A little early, but she's wonderful. Call me when you get in."

Our conversation later went something like this:

"It's a girl. She's so beautiful."

"What's her name?"

"Adelyn Ruth. She's so beautiful."

"What name? Say that again."

"She's so beautiful. Adelyn Ruth, after my mother who was Ruth Adelyn. She's so beautiful."

"How's Ann?"

"She's fine. You've just got to see the baby. She's so beautiful."

"How big is she."

"She's so beautiful. Five and a half pounds, I think. I can't believe it. She's so tiny and so wonderful and so beautiful. They had to throw me out of the hospital tonight."

If this conversation sounds familiar to you, so will many of the things you will read in this book. When we ran the series in *Baby Talk,* we received calls and letters from readers who exclaimed how similar their own experience had been and how comforting the articles were. In addition to Ann and Nevin's experiences, you'll also read commentary from a pediatrician and a child development specialist.

The first year with a first baby is a real eye-opener, literally and figuratively. Whatever their ages, it's the year parents themselves really grow up. Ann and Nevin Kishbaugh went through their first year with Addie Ruth, absorbed all the experiences and emerged as slightly different people. Ann is much more confident in herself and quite comfortable as a mother. Her ability to adjust, sometimes easily, has proven very helpful in her new parenting role. If anything, Nevin is even more philosophical, more willing—and able—to try to figure out what this life is all about. I like them even better as parents than I did before they had Addie.

You will change, too, as you bring up your baby and I feel sure this book will sustain you through the difficult first year. There are times when wrestling alligators looks like more fun than parenting. There are agonizing moments of uncertainty and exhausted moments of sheer frustration. But best of all, there are countless moments of incomparable joy, times when you are sure your baby is a gift beyond compare, without doubt the most beautiful thing ever to appear on this earth. Ann and Nevin cover them all, the highs and the lows, and help first-time parents understand that they are not alone. I think you'll be glad they were open and brave enough to share their first-year of parenting with us.

Ann Whelan
Managing Editor
Baby Talk

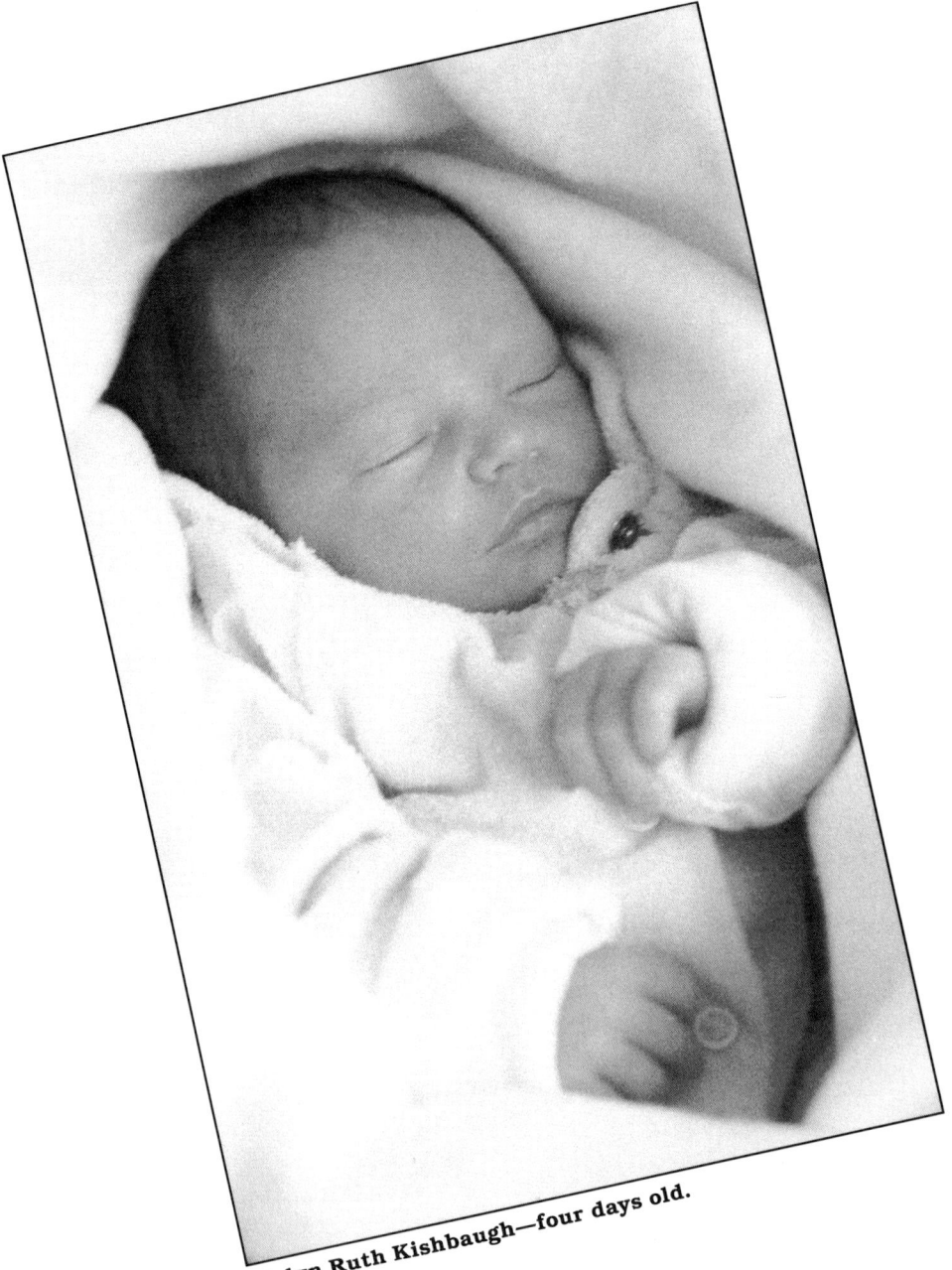

Adelyn Ruth Kishbaugh—four days old.

The Birth

It was your typical middle-of-the-night scenario . . .

Wife: Arghhh (as she is awakened by an enormous contraction and water trickling down her leg).

Uh, honey (shaking him), it's time.

Husband: Gwolfribble . . . Urgh . . . (leaping out of bed) What?

But it was by no means a typical birth, for each experience is unique and special. Ours was particularly memorable because this night happened to be five weeks before our due date. Not that we were totally surprised, Ann had spent the previous five weeks in bed taking ritodrine every four hours to prevent premature labor. But our baby was anxious to be here. So she came with the usual fanfare accorded to such occasions. "Isn't she beautiful?" "Look how tiny her hands and feet are." "Apgars of eight and ten!" Tears. Elation. Relief. She was perfect. She was ours. We had never been happier in our lives.

After the birth, in the initial days of Adelyn's life, many thoughts went through our minds. We had been having these thoughts for quite some time, particularly over the past eight months, but they now began to take more shape and form.

Dad's Thoughts

It's a frightening undertaking—becoming a parent. To be totally responsible for the development of a tiny human being is an intimidating proposition. It has been said that the greatest challenge to the human mind is a blank piece of paper. Not so. The greatest challenge is the blank slate of a newborn. Every action a parent takes has the potential to imprint permanently on the child's psyche; each indelible memory can have a profound effect.

These philosophical thoughts began to occupy my mind from the moment Ann told me she was pregnant. My initial reaction combined both joy and apprehension. What kind of father will I be? Will I remain aware of the importance of my role, or will I let myself become absorbed in the day-to-day monotony, silently relinquishing my ability to influence? How will I answer this child's innocent but persistent questions—with patience and understanding, or with ignorance and frustration?

I was genuinely concerned that I might fail. Fail to guide this little person through the storms and challenges of childhood. Fail to prepare this child for the world outside.

I did not feel ready for the opportunity of parenthood. I still felt too much like a little kid myself.

As the birth of my child became more imminent, my questions changed from "how will I handle this situation" considerations to "what do I want to teach this child?" It was a subtle but important transition. I had become less concerned with specific challenges and more concerned with overall objectives: I want my child to feel loved, to have strong feelings of self-worth, and to show compassion and sensitivity to others. Of course, I still had no idea how to translate these noble aspirations into practice.

I should note here that all this anxiety over my qualifications to be a parent in no way diminished the joy Ann and I felt. In fact, anticipation was felt throughout both of our families, but particularly by my mother, Ruth. This would be her first grandchild. My mother had truly enjoyed parenthood, so the prospect of a grandchild delighted her. (I've always imagined that being a grandparent was a lot like being a parent—except, of course, without all the aggravation and responsibility.) Ann's pregnancy was also a significant tonic for my mother; it helped divert her attention from her problem. She was battling cancer. The baby gave her something positive to focus on.

My mother and I often talked about the trials of parenting—the frustrations, the insecurities, and, of course, the joys. "There is no school for parents," she told me. "You do the best you can and learn along the way. You'll do just fine." "Yeah, sure. That isn't much comfort for a frightened father," I replied. She laughed. "Now just relax. You really will do fine."

On September 30, 1989, Annie brought my little girl into this world. Adelyn Ruth must have been in quite a rush to get here because she came five weeks early. Sadly, this was eleven days too late. My mother had passed away on September 19.

Annie was breastfeeding, so my contact with my daughter was more limited than Annie's. I could only hold her, change her, adore her. I couldn't fill her most insistent need. But one morning, only a few days after we brought little Addie Ruth home, Annie had fed her and put her down so she could take a shower. No sooner was Annie in the shower than Addie Ruth started crying uncontrollably. I didn't know what to do. She had been fed, changed, and coddled. What was wrong? As I leaned over her crib, I suddenly remembered one of the things my mother had told me. "You must be relaxed. Handle your baby with confidence, because a child will sense if you are nervous or tense, and that will make things worse." So I picked up my little girl into my arms and, suddenly confident, sang her softly back to sleep.

My mother had been wrong. There *is* a school for parents, and I am just now finding out how gifted a teacher my mother really was.

Mom's Thoughts

Since Adelyn's birth, I feel very scatterbrained. My days now focus exclusively on her wants and needs—and what we will have for dinner. In the small time allotted to me in between these functions, my thoughts drift in wayward fashion. My mind alights on a thought only to be interrupted by Adelyn's cries. I start to contemplate something, and my mind is distracted by what we might need from the store (more baby wipes?) or how I'm going to get the cleaning done or when Adelyn is going to need me next. I begin an idea only to look down and catch Adelyn in a rare smile. My mind veers off its track. I have many thoughts that are very different from my thoughts one year ago. They are the thoughts of a mother.

I must admit I was worried about my role as a mother with a tiny infant. Would the proper motherly instincts kick in? I had never been keen about infants. I was not one of those people who rushed to hold infants. Many of my friends would pronounce gleefully, "Oh, a baby," when a child arrived and run to grab the infant from the mother's arms. I would peer down at the baby from a distance and comment appropriately on the tiny features or the child's resemblance to the father or mother. Infants were OK. I didn't think they were particularly beautiful because they are basically funny-looking creatures. Interesting, yes. Beautiful, not really. Would I form the proper bond with my child? I knew that I loved children when they started talking and responding to me because I was close to my niece and nephews, but a tiny infant?

When Adelyn was placed on top of me after the birth, I was awed. My husband and I examined her tiny features closely. She was beautiful. Later, she was to nurse at my breast as I held her closely in my arms. She was wonderful. Even later, she was to smile in her sleep as I watched her from the crib side. I was in love. I think I will be rushing to hold infants from now on.

We did it. And we did it well, too. I was so proud of her, of myself, of her father. "It" was a girl, and it was right that we have a girl. We had not cared up to the moment she was born, but it seemed so right when we were told. And with this pronouncement came many different feelings.

Oh, the things we could share as mother and daughter. Watching the *Sound of Music* together and weeping uncontrollably at *Edelweiss*. Shopping and perhaps sharing clothes. Being best friends when she turns twenty and I turn fifty-one.

I also realized that I would have more fears and concerns for a girl child. I know about growing up as a girl and becoming a woman. It is a wonderful thing, but there is much pain and heartache along the way. Appearance concerns. Adolescent insecurities. Relationships with the opposite sex. When she would hurt, I would also be in deep pain.

This is not to say that it is any easier for boys and men. I just do not know about it as I do for a woman.

Because I grew up with two sisters and Nevin grew up with one brother, I would now become "the expert" on raising a girl. Someday in the distant future, Nevin will turn to me with a panicked look and ask, "Annie, is this behavior normal for a girl?" He will also look to me for guidance on how he should relate to his quirky adolescent. And I am really not sure what I will be able to tell him about that!

Oh, the joys and tribulations of being a girl. Adelyn, you have so much to learn and so much to experience. Please be assured, my little girl child, that we will prepare you as best as we can.

I am my mother. I was this child. This thought has occurred to me often since Adelyn was born. I watch her nursing and clutching my finger in her tiny hand. I sit up with her during her "fussy" periods feeling frustrated and angry that she cannot tell me what it is she needs. I watch her sleep and think that she is the most precious gift that I have ever received. For the first time, I feel that I know what my mother went through in raising me. The years of hard work are compensated by the pure joy that is felt at having brought a new life into the world. We are tied together forever. My mother and I. My daughter and I. It is a wonderful life.

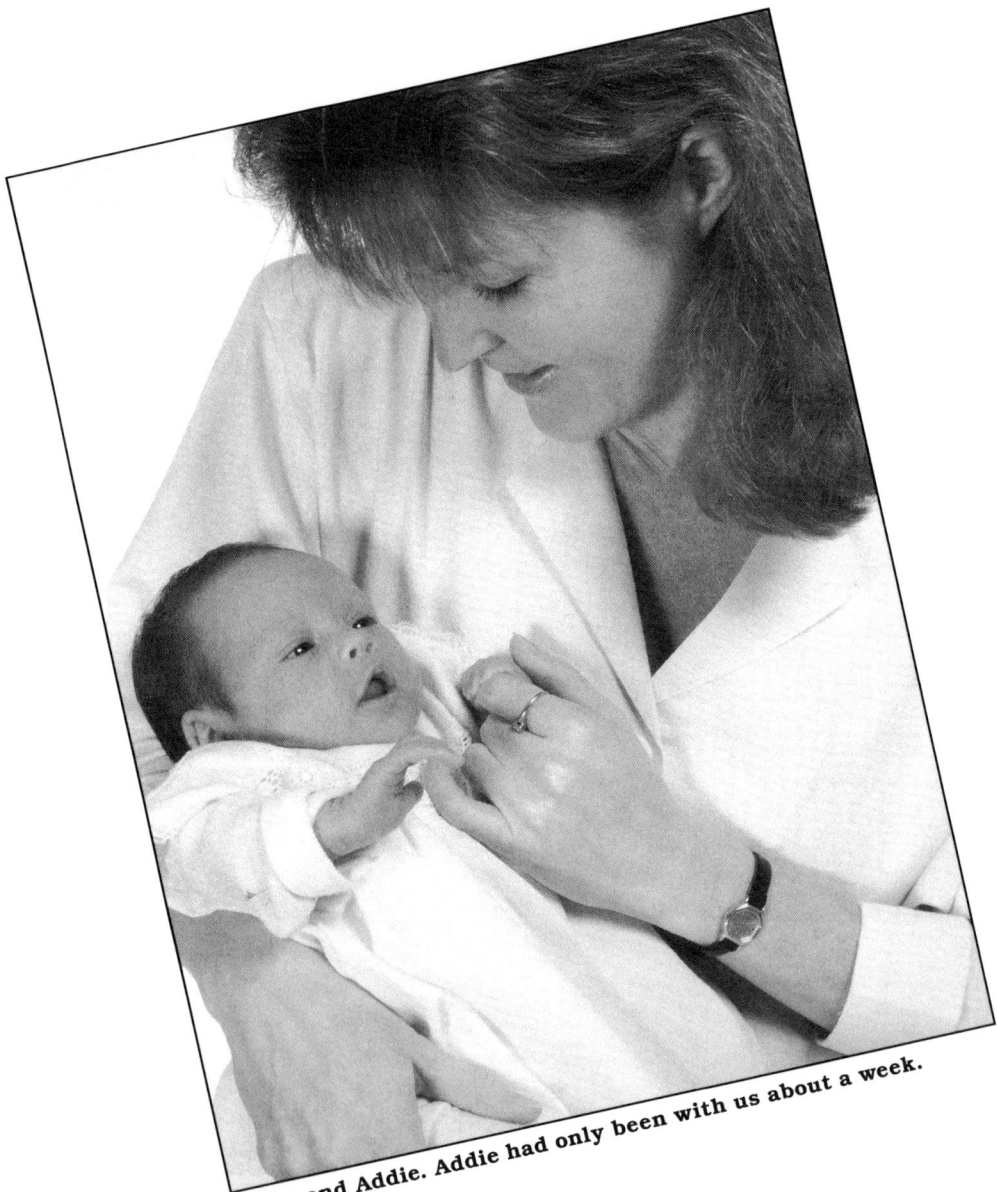

Annie and Addie. Addie had only been with us about a week.

First Month

Mom's Thoughts

Well, here we are—the three of us. Now what do we do?

"Nevin, what does it say in the book about . . . ?"

"Hello, Mom? Sorry to wake you but Adelyn . . ."

"Sis, do you have a minute? Remember when David was . . ."

I must confess. I miss the hospital. Nurses brought the baby in, nurses took the baby away. Meals came, meals went. I dozed. I awakened. I was in pain, yes, but I was exhilarated nonetheless. I knew exactly what to expect at each hour. Nurses fussed about in that happy way that nurses in maternity wards do. They had taken care of me, and they had primarily taken care of my baby. Adelyn Ruth (the name still rolls oddly off the tongue) is so tiny and so fragile, and now she is counting on me to take care of her in the correct way. Me, who knows absolutely nothing about babies. But I will learn. For her sake, I will learn.

I feel so unprepared because with all the events of the previous month (especially the death of Nevin's mother, who was also my dear friend) and now with the early birth of Adelyn, I have not yet gotten a chance to read my books on child care. When we first came home from the hospital, our emotions were reeling, and the house was in total chaos. Adelyn's room wasn't even finished, my mother was in the process of painting the crib, and who knew when the house was last cleaned? I hadn't even seen the first floor in five weeks because I had been bedridden to the second floor! We were two very nervous parents (another foreign word).

The first week was miraculously easy. All Addie Ruth did was sleep and eat. Sleep and eat. (I guess that is all I would have done if I had just experienced the journey she had.) We peeked constantly into her crib. We examined her tiny little body with excruciating detail. We finished her room. My mother came by to help. We began to relax a little. This is easy, we thought. We expounded on Adelyn's virtues to friends who called or dropped by. They gave us a sardonic smile. Then it hit—"Monster baby night." Perhaps I should explain to the uninitiated.

When Adelyn was about two weeks old, there came a day when she seemed to dislike us intensely, and we were not enamored of her in our usual fashion. Even the weather was miserable. It all started about 4:00 P.M. Addie wailed nonstop. Breastfeeding was the only thing that would soothe her. She breastfed continuously for three hours. I was in the midst of the "baby blues" and cried at my failure as a mother.

Nevin stood on the sidelines wringing his hands because he could not feed his daughter, and he could not comfort her mother. Occasionally, he stepped in to give me needed breaks from her wailing. This scenario continued until about 1:00 A.M. Nevin had just finished his shift and was catching a little sleep when I appeared at his bedside with the wailing Addie and said, "You must go out and find some formula. I can't breastfeed anymore." So off he drove with bleary eyes into the miserable night in search of formula.

The story has a happy ending. I found Nevin a little while later back in the kitchen boiling bottles and heating formula like a pro. I made myself a cup of tea and sipped and sniffled while holding Addie, who continued to cry in fits and spurts. A look passed between Nevin and me. When Addie was given the bottle, she gulped furiously. After finishing four ounces, she dropped into a deep, peaceful sleep. Another look passed between us.

Later, we sat in the kitchen congratulating ourselves and feeling our confidence as parents returning. We had discovered what she needed. It felt good. We really were parents. The first test had been passed with a B+, but next time we might get an A. At her bedside later, we stood marveling at her. We quickly forgot the past ten hours of hell. We *still* loved her; nothing she would ever do could change that.

It was the first of many realizations, but we emerged stronger, and it prepared us for the many nights yet to come. We knew we could survive anything together. It would never be as bad as that first time. Our parenting instincts were developing. It was a rite of passage for all of us.

That was one of the times I wish Adelyn had come with directions. I'm sure most new parents feel that way sometimes. Although Adelyn didn't come with directions, she did come with an apnea monitor. I, particularly, have had a hard time adjusting to it. When I first saw her attached to it, my reaction was denial. I cried my heart out for my little "robot" baby. It was very disturbing at first to see her hooked with wires to a box of little flashing lights and to carry a machine on one shoulder as I cradled her in my arm on the other side. The CPR classes deeply disturbed me, and I barely listened to the subsequent monitor class because I was in such a state of shock. When we left the hospital the first day without our child, I was angry. The monitor seemed unnecessary and sadistic. Nevin patiently explained the obvious: Better safe than sorry.

And so we arrived home the following day with our bundle of joy and our bundle of wires. During the first month, we have barely left her room. I have felt tied to this machine and resent the claustrophobia for both of us. Recently, however, I talked with a friend who also had a "monitor baby," and I realized that we could be mobile. I was surprised to learn that my ever-cautious friend had not always taken the machine with her when she left the house. She was with her child so there was no need. I have become braver, traveling first downstairs and then on a few short outings without the monitor. With increased freedom, I can now accept its necessity, and I no longer feel that "something is wrong with this picture."

Despite my various reactions toward this machine, when I was first told Adelyn would need one, I did not panic. A couple of our friends had had babies on the monitor, and I was familiar with it through them. Their support has been invaluable. They are very helpful with tips and have talked with me about my concerns. They have even offered to baby-sit. (That is one of the big problems: finding qualified baby sitters who know CPR. My parents kindly took classes so they could help us out.) Our little support group is wonderful for us, and we don't feel the need to attend our monitor company's meetings. I would, however, highly recommend them to others. It's vital to your mental health to talk about your concerns with others who have had or are having this experience, and the exchange of information can be very valuable.

You might note here that I am doing an awful lot of crying. I am. I don't know exactly why. I just do. I have seen the term "baby blues" numerous times, but I never really gave it much attention. My sister wisely counseled me on its impact when I was in the hospital. "You'll find yourself crying over the stupidest things. Don't let it get to you. If you feel like crying, just cry. It's normal. You're not losing your mind. Call me if you need me." I cry at the drop of a hat now. (And I'm the only one of my teen-age friends who didn't cry during *Love Story* in the 1970s.) Nevin tells me we're out of bread. I cry. A favorite song comes on while Addie is breast-feeding. I cry. We pull adhesive electrodes off of Addie's tender skin. She wails. I cry buckets (and make Nevin do it from now on). It's unnerving to say the least, but like any good cry, it feels good after the moment passes. Nevin has been very supportive and helpful. I had warned him about this, and I think that just the realization that it might happen has helped us through this transition.

In this first month, I am trying particularly hard to take good care of myself. I take naps every day while Addie naps and eat well for both of us. I talk with friends frequently. I accept help when it is offered. I try not to worry about how the house looks. My biggest effort (besides taking care of Addie) is willing my body—and mind—back to its former self. I tell myself that this is only temporary—this pain will go away, I will stop crying, I will become proficient in parenting. For now, I think I'll just concentrate on taking care of me. I need to do this for both Addie and Nevin. I know they'll understand.

Dad's Thoughts

OK, guys, let's face it: in the first few weeks after the baby comes home from the hospital, we get about as much attention as a third-string offensive lineman on an 0–12 team. I'm not saying we're unimportant; the truth is, we're vital. But for the first few weeks, we're on the sidelines. The real action is between Mother and Child, and rightly so.

When Adelyn was born on that sunny September morning, I kind of felt like I was speeding through a glass tunnel. I could only focus on those things that were directly

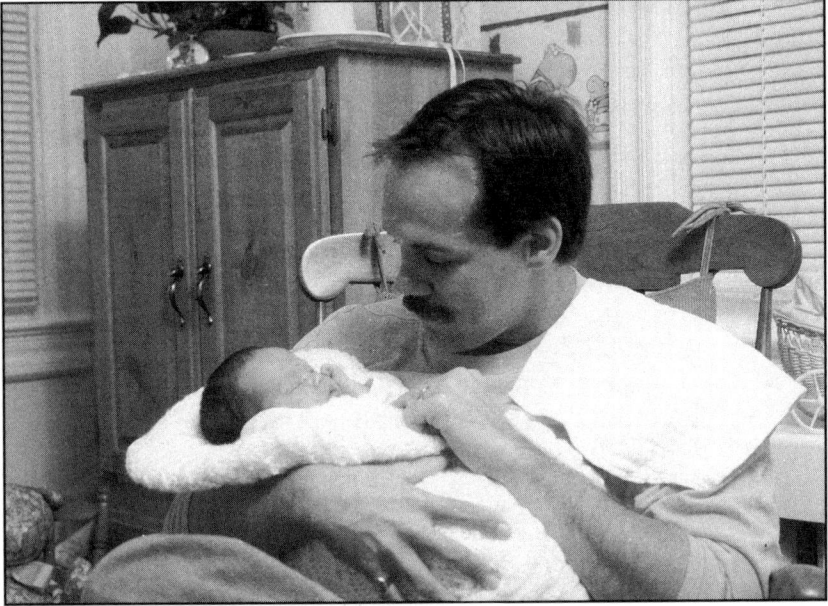

Here I am, trying to look like I know what I'm doing. The fact that she's sound asleep helps me pull it off.

in front of me, everything else being reduced to a shapeless blur. There was so much to do. My daughter was five weeks early, her room wasn't even ready yet, I had to spread the news to family and friends, and I hadn't slept in two days. That last part was by far the least of my worries—the day my girl was born, I had so much adrenalin pumping through my system, I could have run a marathon on my hands.

But, when Mother and Child come home, we fathers become support personnel. Basically, we do those tasks that allow our wives to concentrate their attention on the baby. At this point, my primary responsibility is to help make Ann's life easier. This is a rough time for her. For the last nine months, she's been carrying a lot of weight (both literally and figuratively), and delivery probably takes more out of a woman than any man realizes. Like many women these days, Annie is breastfeeding, so no matter how much I may be willing, I cannot even relieve her from the middle-of-the-night feedings—which would allow her to get some much-needed, uninterrupted sleep.

So I do what I can—help with the house, the shopping, the laundry. As for the baby, well, there's not much I can do. I change her sometimes and get up at 3:00 A.M. if the monitor alarm goes off, but, for the most part, I'm left out of the picture. "Monster baby night" changed the scenario a little, but I still feel like I'm on the periphery. I guess what bothers me most about all this is that I cannot have the same relationship with my daughter that my wife has. They are infinitely closer by means of biology, and that fundamentally changes the relationship—at least for now.

On our first wedding anniversary, three years ago, a close friend of ours gave us a gift of two small books—the pages, blank. Given our backgrounds in writing and editing, they were the perfect gifts. They were misplaced until about a year ago, when Ann found them hidden in a bookcase. Their resurfacing has turned out to be fortuitous. They now provide me with the means to communicate with my infant daughter. They will become, I hope, a highly valued legacy to her.

About a month before I found out Annie was pregnant, I began writing essays in my book. My mother was in the midst of her battle with cancer, and I wanted to keep some notes about her ordeal and her remarkable strength and courage. I really don't know why I began to write in the book. I had no audience except myself, but maybe that would have been enough.

Then I discovered that Annie was pregnant, and suddenly I was writing *to* someone. I had an audience. I would still write about my mother's grave challenge, but my focus had widened considerably. The essays, addressed to my as yet unborn child, became letters, a format I was more comfortable with.

I write to my daughter on any subject that appeals to me—from family history to current events. It is, I guess, my way of connecting with her. I have tried to convey all the

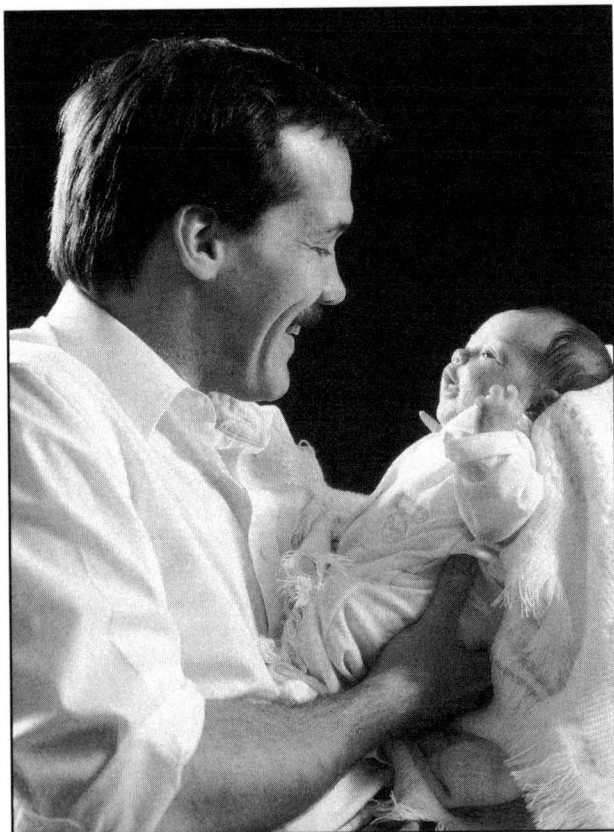

When she is old enough to understand, I may not remember exactly how it felt to look at her or hold her.

promise I see in this tiny newborn, how much she has to look forward to in her life, and how much joy she has brought to us already. I hope these letters will be important to her. I hope they will tell her something about me, about how much she means to both of us. When she is old enough to understand, I may not remember exactly how it felt just to look at her or hold her. When she is old enough to understand, I may have forgotten all I wanted to say, or worse, I may not be here.

First Month—Pediatric Commentary by Dr. Marie Keith

The first month! It's a tough time. I found the schedule more demanding than my internship. You never seem to catch up on your sleep. Fear and anxiety must co-exist with the pure love new babies bring to a family. Your world changes dramatically.

Experiencing all this just after a family death and with an apnea monitor can stretch couples in ways they hadn't thought possible. In many respects, Ann and Nevin are typical of the young parents I see in my practice. But like all couples, they are special in their own way.

It's not all that unusual that little Addie Ruth was sent home with an apnea monitor. Premature infants often do not have much stability in their autonomic nervous system, which controls heart rate and breathing. Though premature, Addie arrived very close to being ready for life. Ann's five weeks in bed on ritodrine gave the baby invaluable time to develop almost to a fully mature stage.

But when the infant was observed immediately after birth, physicians were concerned about her low heart rate, so Addie had a test called a pneumogram, which showed respiratory slowing with a resulting low heart rate. So she was given an apnea monitor that she will remain attached to during sleep until she is about six months old, at which point problems stemming from an unstable autonomic nervous system are resolved.

The complete physical exam babies are given shortly after birth helps us gauge a newborn's relative health and take care of any problems or abnormalities in a timely manner. Some things need to be done immediately; others can wait or are better done at a later date. Aside from the need for an apnea monitor, Addie passed her exam with flying colors.

Pediatricians also can't help but take some measure of the new parents. We see them at a very special time—they're thrilled and relieved but we usually can sense their fear and apprehension about knowing what to do for this new life and when to do it.

I tell them they can't know everything they need to know on day one. Parents learn every day. As the baby communicates her needs, parents respond and learn. Also, most new parents buy a few baby care books which provide a measure of security.

I especially liked some of the things Ann and Nevin had to say about their experiences with Addie. Nevin said his mother taught him to learn from the baby, which couldn't be more true. If you pay attention, you'll always learn from your baby. Ann saw the continuity from mother to child. We rarely sense this important aspect of life until we become parents ourselves.

It's a good thing the rigors of the first month and the uncertainties of a new life are so enmeshed with wonder and joy and love. While few of us might wish to repeat that demanding time, we might like to put just a bit of the consummate joy into each day of our lives. As Ann says, and as I see every day, it's a wonderful life.

First Month—Child Development Commentary by Dr. Anita Hurtig

Appropriately during these first weeks of the baby's life, Ann and Nevin are focusing on issues of their own feelings—apprehension, expectations, excitement. Their sensitivity to their essential role in the baby's development is a hallmark of good parenting.

D. W. Winicott, a British pediatrician and keen observer of infant development, noted that "there is no such thing as a baby." What he meant was that a baby only exists as part of a unit, tied through constant interaction, even before birth, to its mother, and to father, too, as Nevin's poignant account of his calming Addie illustrates. Nevin reveals both the grandiosity of the parents' estimate of the baby's vulnerability to parental failure, but also the realistic awareness that parents can and must have "profound" effects on the development of the child's psyche.

Infant developmental research has provided us with increasingly persuasive evidence that babies are remarkably responsive to even the most seemingly subtle parental behaviors, including handling, vocalizing, and glancing. Ann's feelings and concerns reflect the natural uncertainties which any mother brings to the wonder of giving birth, of having a part of oneself, felt but unseen, become separate and external.

Ann asks, "Would I form the proper bond with my child?" What does it mean "to bond?" Is it a process that automatically occurs with motherhood, or a complex process of interaction that fosters meaningful attachment?

Ann's awe, patience and pride, and her joy in the process of regeneration, all point to a capacity for attachment. But the task of attachment is an interactive process. Adelyn is not just the recipient of her mother and father's love and attention. She impacts on them, and so her capacity to respond plays no small part in the attachment process. As we follow Addie and her parents over the next twelve months, we will see how her development, particularly given the hazards of premature birth, allows us to observe the subtle dance of life that baby, mother, and father choreograph as an ensemble.

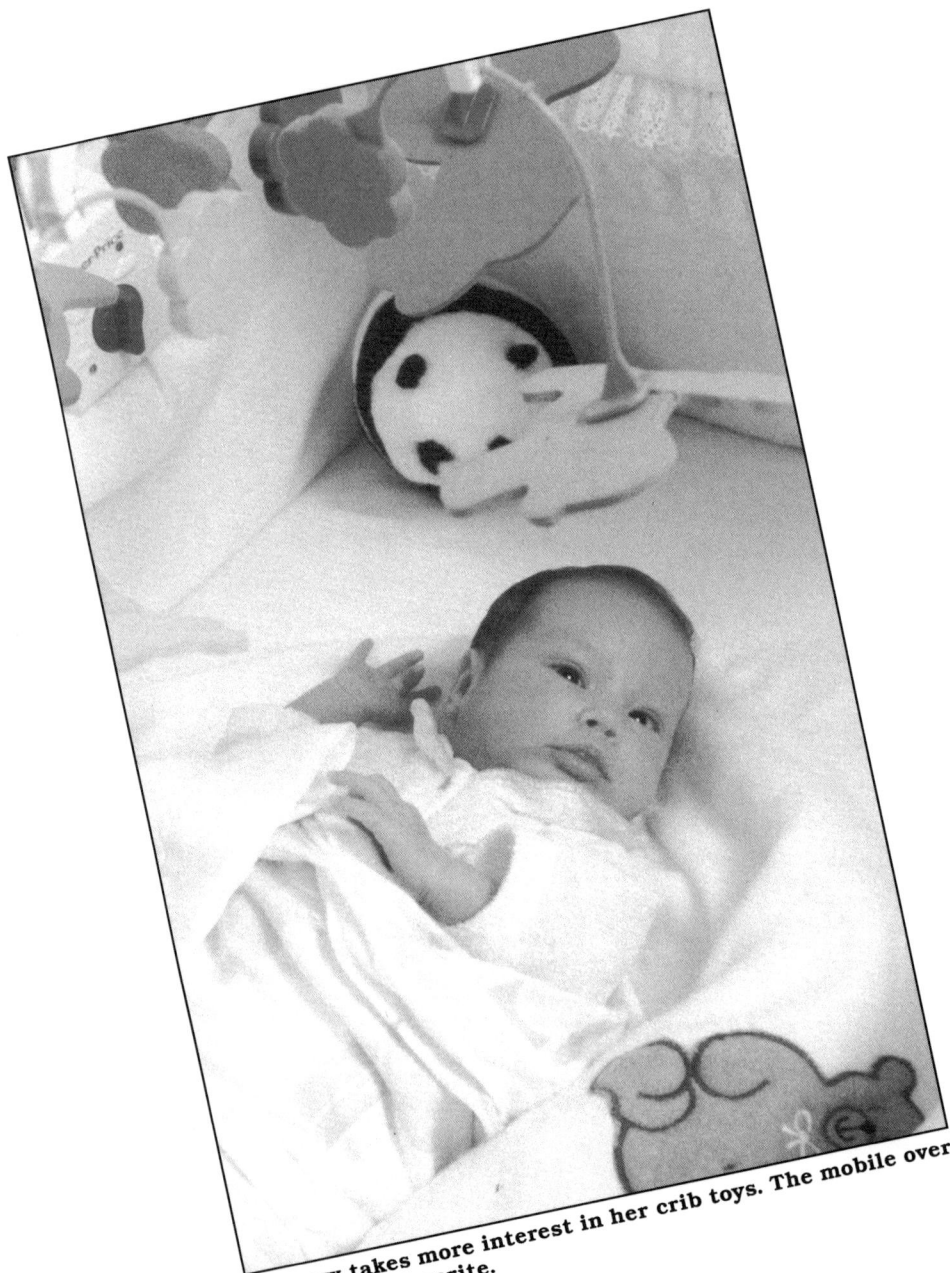

She now takes more interest in her crib toys. The mobile over her crib is a favorite.

Second Month

Mom's Thoughts

Addie and I might be beginning to understand one another. I stress *might* because we still take each day at a time. I know some things about her now that I did not understand during our first month together. For example, she may cry out and fuss over a bowel movement, but that doesn't mean I need to run to her rescue. She likes to be kept as warm as possible when I change her diaper. She hates being put on my shoulder when gas is distressing her. She likes a long cuddle before her last nightly feeding. I can amuse her for half-hour periods, but she then gets bored and needs to relax. I think we may be getting along. At the very least, we have reached detente.

When I think back on that first month, we were strangers in a strange land. We have all made progress. Addie is much more secure in our world, and we are much more secure about answering her needs. Oh, there are still those days when our lines of communication (such as they are) get garbled, but we're learning—with every day we are learning.

Our biggest coping mechanism at this time is learning to think from Adelyn's vantage point. It's not easy and doesn't come naturally. We had to drop all knowledge of what we knew of life and consider ourselves as aliens visiting for the first time. I have found that anyone who has had experience with infants summons this psychology when discussing infant care.

You're not born with patience. It is learned. That has been my mantra during the difficult times. I thought I was patient. I've found that I am not, but I am learning. Addie is learning, too. Our newly found patience has helped us develop a crucial list of comforting tricks for fussy periods when we know all of Adelyn's physical needs have been met:

1. Wrap her gently and tightly in one or two blankets.

2. Help her find her thumb. (Some may prefer a pacifier.)

3. Hold her on my shoulder while rubbing her back gently. Ignore rooting sounds in my ear.

4. Put on music and sing loudly while rocking or walking around the house.

5. Lay her on my chest and gently talk and rub her back rhythmically (very successful!).

6. March like a soldier while cradling her in my arms or jiggling her.

7. Rub her back while playing a musical toy if she is fussy but ready to drop off to sleep any minute.

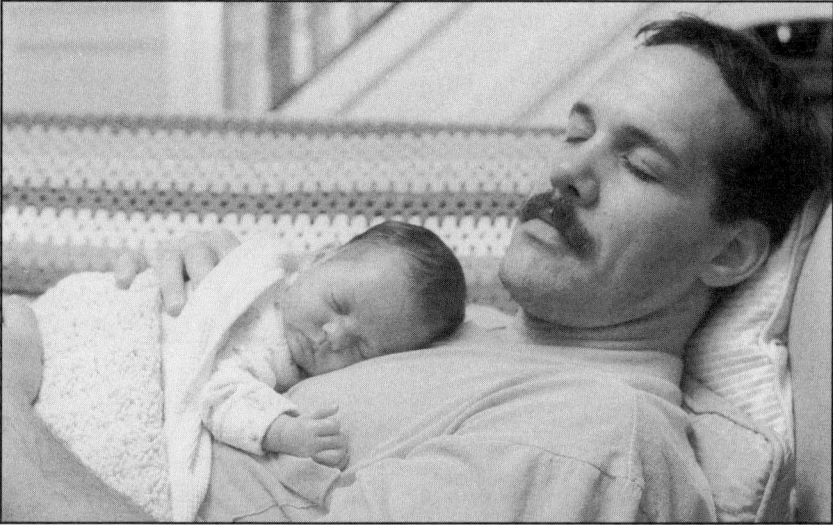

Dad successfully comforts a colicky Addie and gets a nap in the bargain.

8. Cushion her tightly in an infant swing and play Disney music (her favorite) loudly.

9. When all else fails, put on television to keep myself sane.

10. Hand her to her father.

On hearing of our experiences, a good friend sent us *79 Ways to Calm a Crying Baby* (Greene Books—a good shower present). It was a helpful supplement, and both of us leafed through it frantically when our list had been exhausted. The author astutely points out perhaps the most important coping mechanism of all: a sense of humor.

Addie has been described by her pediatricians as "very alert," which, of course, makes us feel very proud that we had a hand in this development. She has always followed voices with her eyes and strains to get her eyes in focus. In this second month, Addie is getting better at making eye contact. When she does, her gaze is surprisingly penetrating. Nevin attributes this to intelligence (typical father, right?); but perhaps she is studying every line in our faces and every movement of our mouths, just as the books say babies do at this stage. As her face is fascinating to us, so we must be to her. We love to watch her. Tongue in. Tongue out. Mouth screwed up like she has sucked a lemon. Mouth open like a bird. Eyes crossed. Eyes connecting with ours. Much more fun than watching television.

I can tell her weight and height have increased dramatically this month, which is common for premature infants. I still remember how light she was when I held her five pounds and six ounces to my breast. Her seven pound, ten ounce frame is now making my arms and back sore. (I'm looking forward to being able to use my hips when her neck is stronger.) It's also getting harder to maneuver her between the arms of the rocker, and we are starting to put away clothes that do not fit her. No wonder she has to sleep a lot!

Addie's head is beginning to stop bobbing at our shoulders and she is able to hold it up herself for several minutes. She still can't raise her head very well when she lays on her abdomen, but she picks it up nicely to move it from side to side when she's looking at the toys in her crib or when she's angry.

Adelyn's little hands seem to have the grip of a vise. When breastfeeding, she latches onto my finger or my shirt like a drowning woman, and when she is angry or upset, she can really squeeze. I am now putting rattles into this eager, searching hand, and she holds them unknowingly for a short time.

Perhaps one of my greatest joys was finding Addie one morning in a different position from the one I had placed her in. She now moves from her side to her back and wiggles herself up to press her head against the bumpers.

Particularly at the end of the second month, we started to see some signs of intelligence developing. Dad received his first real smile one night while holding Addie Ruth and talking softly to her. Mom received one a few days later. It has been my policy not to talk during nightly feedings so Addie can learn the difference between night and day. During the day, the room is bright and I babble incessantly. At night by the light of a dim bulb, I am the silent, smiling Madonna. We do our business, and then we are both off to dreamland after a few cuddles. This policy has been very successful so far, but there was one night when Addie decided to run for Miss Congeniality. It took all of my effort not to respond in kind and finally, while rocking her, I looked down and said, "Miss, you are supposed to be asleep." She looked straight into my eyes with a wide smile that stole my heart.

Adelyn is also taking a lot more interest in her crib toys. The mobile can amuse her for five-minute stretches. A mirror can keep her occupied until sleep overcomes her. The musical toys cause her to perk her ears in interest or may lull her to sleep depending on her mood. Toward the end of this month, a baby gym and her other toys in various combinations (only a few at a time) can amuse her for twenty to thirty minutes. She squeals and kicks her legs in amusement. Mom "talks" back to her like a ventriloquist during these times. (Ever hear the voice of a soft alphabet block or a cotton and polyester panda?)

Adelyn is now awake more, and this has been both gratifying and frustrating. Because she can't do much, it's hard to keep her from getting bored. We go from one amusement to the next. Perhaps some crib time, then a ride in her stroller outside. Reading is reserved for winding down times; however, this has yet to be amusing for very long and is more for Mom than for Adelyn. (I don't know why she doesn't take to *Crime and Punishment.*) Trips to the local mall are usually successful. Lights. Colors. Noises. Movement. At times, however, they can be overly stressful for her. Timing it seems is everything. We went to our first sale together, had a great time in the beginning, and even breastfed very well in a fitting room. But after four hours, Addie got very fussy and had a hard time going down for a nap later. I have been striving for variety and stimulation, but I have to learn to listen to her cues more and remember that she has years of learning ahead. She is, after all, only two months old. (But she has such intelligent eyes!)

Perhaps because of Addie's prematurity, we have had difficult times in the areas of diapering and bathing. The diapering resolved itself with a little help from me. I covered the plastic vinyl of her changing pad with a big, soft terry cloth towel that makes her feel warm and cozy late at night when the temperature is lower. Her one-piece fuzzy sleepers are also easy to maneuver her in and out of while keeping her cozy and warm. My voice and the decorative wall border, which is at her eye level and is covered with animals, provide Addie with necessary distractions from the discomfort of the task at hand. She, too, is growing up.

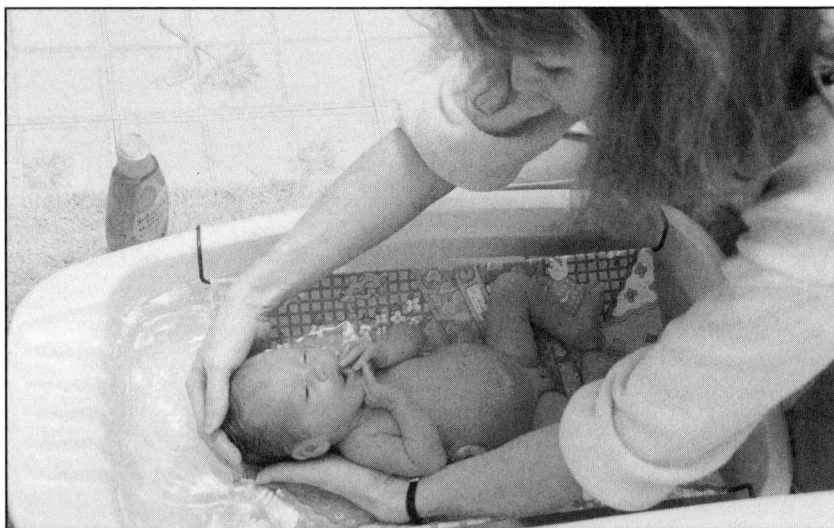

Addie gets her first real bath. You can really see how tiny she is. You can also see that her first bath isn't a source of great joy for her.

Bathing, however, is still a problem. I waited until the second month to give Addie her first bath because she was so distressed at diapering and changing. I was very afraid of her reactions to the bath, and I didn't want to frighten her unnecessarily. The books I'm reading advise that infants do not get really dirty, and cleaning the important little parts daily with wet cotton balls is sufficient. We pursued this course for a while, but people were always asking me how she liked her bath and I felt that perhaps it was I who had the problem, not Addie. I was secretly terrified of bathing her. I thought that I might damage Addie permanently either by dropping or clumsily holding her.

So I read and reread how to give a bath and the day finally came when I decided to take the plunge. I told Nevin, "I need your help this morning with Adelyn's first bath. You read from the book and I'll wash." He eagerly agreed although he wasn't that much help from behind his camera! Surprisingly, that bath went *very* well until we had to leave the bathroom to put on her clothes in her bedroom. She wailed and shook, and I suffered horrible feelings of guilt. Her next bath wasn't until a week later. Addie Ruth is still having problems with this step and has developed a distaste for having her hair washed. Everyone tells me that soon taking a bath will become her favorite activity. Hmmm. I'm waiting patiently for that day.

Because Nevin and I work as freelancers, it was important for us to carefully investigate quality medical coverage that was affordable. We found that there were not a lot of options, but luckily, a health maintenance organization operating in our state met both of our needs. Because our general practitioner was affiliated with this group, it seemed a natural transition for us to subscribe. Since I was very satisfied with my prenatal care, particularly in light of my medical complications (premature labor and high blood pressure during delivery), we were confident that Adelyn's pediatric needs would be taken care of satisfactorily. As with other medical groups, our pediatric care is given by a group practice of three doctors. So far, we've had two of the three doctors and found we are particularly pleased with one pediatrician. We now make it a point to schedule our visits with him.

The nursing staff is very talented and efficient, and they seem truly excited about Adelyn, which is wonderful for a new mother such as me. They have answered our many questions patiently and intelligently and with no negative reaction to our insecurity or, at times, our stupidity. For instance, the first time we called them, we were in a panic because Addie had a hair in her eye. Not exactly crisis material, but Nevin had upset me when he cried out,

"Look, both of her eyes are watery and weeping. What's wrong? Quick, call the clinic." The nurse patiently explained what to do, and the situation was remedied quickly.

Our latest concern has been Adelyn's obsession with her bowel movements. She becomes extremely frustrated with this activity and voices her concerns loudly and with much writhing of her little body. I was very worried that she might hurt herself, but the nurse assured me that this was common and she would come to no harm. After giving me some practical suggestions, the nurse said, "Kids are funny. She may just be developing a dramatic personality." This struck me as very funny, and I now call Adelyn my little actress.

One of the biggest problems that we and others with apnea monitors have is that false alarms do occur and, at times, can be very inconvenient. For example, Adelyn has had very fussy days where she wails at the world angrily for seemingly no reason. At the conclusion of these days, we all fall exhaustingly into sleep only to be awakened by numerous alarms. Adelyn goes into a deep sleep after these fussy periods, and her breathing becomes very shallow. The machine is not sensitive enough to pick up this shallow breathing, so it responds with alarms as though she has stopped breathing. We race into her room and shake her to some level of consciousness. At times, she becomes fully awake, seems scared, and needs to be comforted back to sleep. Needless to say, these experiences can be frustrating, but the old adage again comes to mind: Better safe than sorry. We would, of course, walk over hot coals for this child, so what is a little less sleep?

Adelyn and I are enjoying a good breastfeeding relationship. While it felt awkward at first (body positioning, sore nipples, is she getting enough?), it is now relaxing—yes, even soothing. I feel fortunate that she took so easily and readily to me, especially after being on a bottle for the first two days of life because of my medication for high blood pressure. Although I had made up my mind long ago to breastfeed and had read a little on the subject, I was surprised at how demanding it really is. Being on call every three or four hours is a difficult adjustment. It seemed I would no sooner put her down to sleep and accomplish one task when she would be awake again, ready to eat. I felt terribly unproductive because of this schedule and mentioned this to my sister one day. She was incredulous. "Annie," she said, "you'll never be more productive than you are now." She was right and her insight helps me tremendously when I view my dusty house in disgust.

My favorite time with Adelyn is breastfeeding in the late hours of the night. We are both very sleepy and cold so we cuddle together for warmth, and she tucks her head into the hollow of my neck as I am burping her. It is heaven. I will miss these times when she eventually sleeps through the night, although I will enjoy sleeping deeply again. There are signs now that she will soon give up this late feeding. A few times this month she has slept for six- and seven-hour periods. I have been startled awake on those occasions and panicked that something was wrong. I have quickly become accustomed to this new way of life—and I kind of like it.

It has been a critical month for developing a new "normal" lifestyle for Nevin and me. Life revolves around Addie, but we are fitting her into our daily lives and routines. While we spent the first month in her room, in the second month we are visiting friends and relatives, performing necessary household chores with her in her carriage not far from us, switching off child care duties as one of us needs the time for our work, and learning how best to take her with us as we run errands. She adds another dimension to our life as a couple. Nevin and I especially savor our time together. When we get it, it's far sweeter than it ever was. It feels like stolen time, and we have learned to use it more wisely. Conversations are broader, and our discussions are decidedly far-ranging. The future of our little girl is prominent in our thoughts. It is no longer me and him against the world, it is our family at stake. We act more cautiously.

So many things are much more clear to us now. What our parents went through. What friends have experienced. We understand the fragility of life. Life before Adelyn is getting harder and harder to imagine. She is here. We feel complete.

Dad's Thoughts

With so much going on in our lives during the last two months—specifically the wonder of Adelyn's birth and the trauma of my mother's death—it is only now that I have the time to talk about a remarkable transition men make. I'm talking about the move from "married man" to "family man." It is a genuine metamorphosis—as momentous a change as from boyhood to manhood. The evidence of the transition, however, is not external. It is internal; it is a radical change of perspective.

Women, I'm sure, undergo something similar—perhaps even more profound. But their transition is more gradual. It begins first with the psychological understanding that they carry in them a new life. As the pregnancy develops and the physical signs become more obvious, so does the change in perspective.

The change for me occurred, or should I say I became aware of the change, when Annie came home from the hospital after having gone into premature labor four days before. It was the end of August, and the baby wasn't due for another ten weeks. We were told that the situation was common and the pregnancy would continue normally provided Ann stayed in bed for the duration and continued taking the medication they had used in the hospital to stop the premature contractions. The medication was called ritodrine and was administered every four hours. It belongs to a class of drugs known as anti-abortives—an ominous and unpleasant sounding description, if you ask me. (Euphemisms abound in our society. You'd think that with pregnant couples being nervous enough they could come up with a description that sounds less violent—maybe something like enduro-term).

When Ann came home from the hospital, she came with a twenty-hour supply of the medication. We had been cautioned at the hospital that the medication must be taken every four hours—on time every time—or the contractions could start again.

The next afternoon, around 4:00 P.M., I went, with prescription in hand, to our local pharmacy. Ann had taken her last pill at 2:00 P.M., so I had a full two hours before her next dose was due.

The pharmacist took the prescription, and I sat down to wait. Ten or fifteen minutes went by, and I went to the counter to ask how much longer.

"This prescription for Kishbaugh," the woman at the counter asked the pharmacist, "how much longer?"

He sifted through a small pile of prescriptions on his desk, found it and read it. (I presume for the first time.)

"I don't think we have it," he said.

"What?"

"I don't think—"

"No, no," I interrupted, "I heard you. *Why* don't you have it?"

"There's not much call for this," he explained. "It's an anti-abortive."

There was that word again. The sound of it made me feel uneasy.

"We can probably get it for you, though," he went on.

"When?"

"Tomorrow."

"Forget it."

I took the prescription back, genuinely annoyed that I had to wait around a full fifteen minutes before they determined that the medication wasn't on their shelves.

I got back in the car and headed for another pharmacy. It hadn't occurred to me that a particular medication wouldn't be in stock. That had never happened before. I guess we're all somewhat spoiled in that regard. We function under the assumption that when we go into a store, especially a drug store, the item we're looking for will be there, available.

At the second drug store, I handed the prescription over

and asked that they check to see if it was in stock. It was nearing 5:00 P.M. and I didn't want to lose time waiting for nothing.

They didn't have it either.

It was at this point that I noticed the change. I was no longer annoyed at the inconvenience, I was angry. It was the type of anger you feel when you are threatened—a cold, determined anger. But the difference was that I was not the one being threatened—my wife and child were. I also noticed that fear was not a component of my emotions the way it might have been if I were the vulnerable one. Such fear, I guess, is the result of some uncertainty, the prospect of failure. And, in this instance, failure was not an option. Whether or not it was true, I felt that the life of my child was at genuine risk.

As I approached the counter of the third pharmacy, I ignored the other patrons waiting and stuck the prescription under the pharmacist's nose.

"Do you have this?" I asked.

"I-I don't know. I'll have to check."

The poor guy was a little taken aback, I suppose. I don't like to be rude, and I get annoyed when others are. But, time was running short, and to tell the truth, I really didn't care.

No, he didn't have it either. At this point, time was too short to go running around through traffic. The only smart thing to do was to use the phone. I called a nearby drug store. They didn't have it either, but their other store might. If so, they would call me back.

A few minutes later, I got the call. Their other store did have the medicine in stock, and they could transfer it in half an hour.

I walked into the house at five minutes to six, ritodrine in hand. I was truly grateful to that last pharmacist. He had put everything else on hold to make sure I got that prescription. I walked up the stairs to the bedroom quite casually. (Hey, I had a whole five minutes to spare.)

Ann looked at me funny when I walked in.

"What took you so long?" she asked.

"Oh, um, they were a little crowded."

Second Month—Child Development Commentary by Dr. Anita Hurtig

It is a source of constant wonder to observant parents that babies can change so dramatically from month to month in the first year of life. What Annie and Nevin are responding to in these first two months is Addie's awakening as a "feeling" entity. They are sensitive to the fact that even as early as two months, and even though she was a premature baby, Addie is sensitive to sound, to touch, to movement, and to position. Most telling is their awareness that intensity is the crucial determinant of how stimulating any of these sensations can be. While infants respond to rising stimulation and excitation, this stimulation can't be too intense or it becomes stressful. If the stimulation is too mild the baby is non-responsive; if too intense, the baby withdraws. Finding this optimal level is part of the "dance" of interaction. Ann recognizes that Addie has her own very particular level of responsivity, which Ann identifies as "signs of intelligence." How wonderful to have a parent see the mutual balancing of responses as a sign of the baby's intelligence, a parent's way of understanding that the baby is developing a sense of the relationship between herself and her mother, or father, with pleasure and comfort rewarded for both. This relationship between the baby's state of internal satisfaction and her gaze at her mother or father's face is crucial, for it becomes the matrix for later associations which permit feelings of nurturing and intimacy to follow.

A large part of Ann and Nevin's concerns in these first two months are the very special needs of a premature baby, vulnerable to breathing distress and therefore requiring an apnea monitor. All parents dream of the perfect baby, the chance to redo any imperfections they see in themselves. Ann describes how important it is for parents to be able to reach out and utilize support from medical personnel and personal friends. She also describes how essential it is that parents find a way to normalize their lives as soon as possible, particularly considering their own needs as a couple, as well as parents. Ann and Nevin have been sensitive to each other's needs, which are for Nevin to feel important in his role as father and for Ann to get some relief from child care so that she can feel productive in other aspects of her life. The very fact that they are able to comfortably share these responsibilities in Addie's first two months makes the demands of the coming years seem less anxiety-provoking.

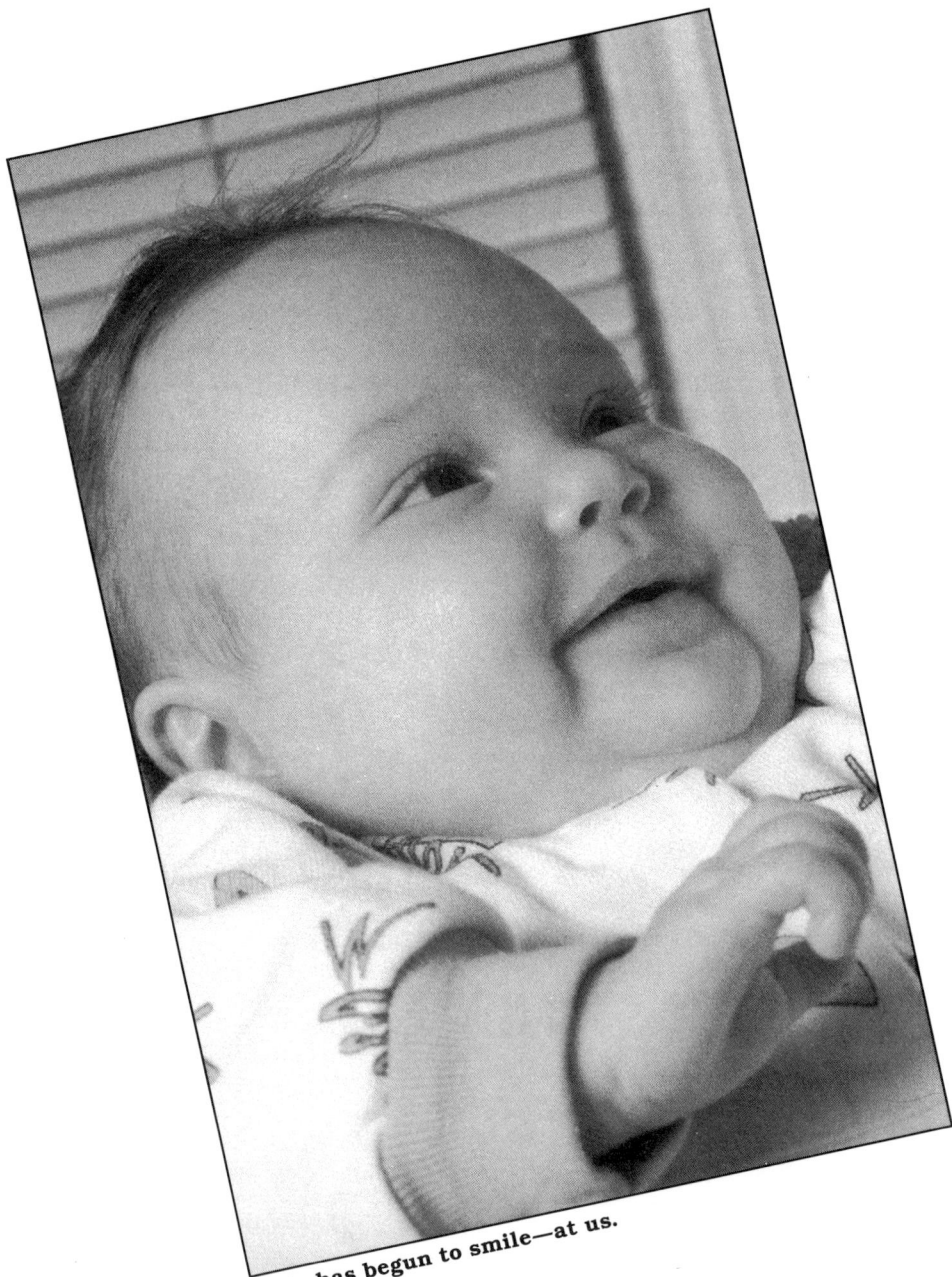

Addie has begun to smile—at us.

Third Month

Mom's Thoughts

Adelyn began her third month rather unhappily. At her two-month checkup, she received her first DPT shot and the oral polio vaccine. Addie screamed in horror at the first and tried to spit out the second. It was a trying moment in her short life, but after all the excitement, she fell into a deep sleep.

In general, however, our visit was very satisfactory. The pediatrician was pleased with her progress: Addie was gaining weight nicely, and she had had no low heart alarms in the last month. He warned me that the DPT shot could cause the apnea monitor to go off a lot that night and prescribed Infant's Tylenol® for any discomfort. Addie experienced neither. She was perhaps a little fussy, but it would be hard to distinguish that from her normal night-time behavior.

At the end of the visit, our pediatrician asked questions relating to her development. When he asked whether we had started receiving a lot of smiles, I sadly reported that we had only gotten a few.

Mom and Dad, on the other hand, began the month happily. We had our first night out. Grandma offered to baby-sit, and knowing we should never turn down an offer such as that, we eagerly made plans. Since my parents knew infant CPR, we were assured Addie would be in very good hands.

I planned my day around our night out making sure Addie's feeding time fell just when we arrived at my parent's house so we would have four glorious hours to ourselves. (Addie is still on a four-hour feeding schedule with slight variations, which makes it easier for me to plan my day; sometimes, however, she still surprises me.) I also had to plan getting her ready, getting her things ready, and getting me ready.

It wasn't easy, but I was excited and it was well worth it for a night out. Luckily, I had thought ahead and picked out an outfit that would fit my still-changing figure and allow me to breastfeed easily. (I have found that most of my nicer outfits and dresses are not made for breastfeeding, unfortunately.) Nevin grinned when he saw me. A real change from big sweat suits! We had a wonderful time being out among adults (we did call home once, though), and my parents and Addie had fun, too.

This month, we have seen significant changes. The infant we took care of at the beginning of the month seemed an entirely different child than the baby who emerged at the end. The third month began much the same as the second ended: Her fussy periods or "colic" continued to baffle and frustrate us. But just after Nevin commented, "I can't wait until she ends this stage," one morning this wonderful baby appeared. The first signs were physical. Eyelashes—long and luxurious (the kind women die for)—came overnight. Pudgy, round, full cheeks grew suddenly. Pudgy little fingers and pudgy little legs completed the package. Her legs straightened out. Drool flowed from the corners of her mouth.

And best of all, those big, toothless grins that doctor had asked about came with devastating force. She loved us after all. She knew who we were at last! I duly noted the change on her first-year calendar: "Smiles—lots of them." We were actually able to prompt them. "Cootchie, cootchie, coo." Grin. "How's daddy's little girl." Grin. We were ecstatic.

In addition, her attention span got longer. She would lie and kick her legs in delight over her mobile for forty minutes. She loved looking around from her swing. We propped her in an infant seat (cushioning her tightly) next to us while we read the paper or watched television. She actually was happy just watching the activity in the room. We were thrilled. She would watch us intently. We would talk to her. She would doze off and awaken again. She was happy!

With this change in her personality, I was now able to establish some semblance of routine. Morning playtime with her mobile and a few choice toys for thirty to forty minutes would tire her out until noon. Propping her in an infant seat and taking her from room to room as I cleaned kept her quiet, happy, and best of all, distracted from the bowel problems she had been having. She catnapped cheerfully. Evenings were still a bit unsettled, but they were not the true colic we had experienced before. Some play, followed by a bath and feeding, would wind her down nicely for bed. I have found that she will not go to sleep in her crib unless it is night, which is as it should be.

These changes are gratifying. My head is swelling with my feelings of success as a mother and my confidence that I can "read" my child. (Who is bringing up whom here?) She is sending me signals ("I don't want to do this anymore." "I want to sleep now." "I want you to play with me."), and I am able to pick them up, most of the time.

The telltale sign that we are forming a strong bond came one day when we were in a store. The line was long; tensions were high. Wails started sounding from her stroller. I looked around nervously. The wails grew louder. Somehow I switched the packages from my arms to the stroller and replaced them with a tearful Addie. I began rocking and murmuring. The crying stopped. She then looked around. I was so proud. I was her mom. She was my daughter. All the people in line knew it too.

When Adelyn was ten weeks old, I awoke one morning in answer to her call with a pounding headache. I stumbled into her room, leaned into her crib, and picked her up. She felt like a fifty-pound weight. I was even further surprised when she latched onto my left breast. I almost screamed from the pain. Somehow I persevered through her feeding, gritting my teeth with each sucking motion. The right breast was fine, thank goodness, but as she fed I felt my temperature rising. I prayed she would go down for a nap after her feeding.

Luckily, I had glanced over the section on breast infections in my breastfeeding book, and I had a sneaky suspicion that was what I had. I quickly located the book. My symptoms were on target. The first instruction was, "Go immediately to bed." I took the book to bed and nudged Nevin awake. "I feel rotten," I said and began to read to him from the book. The next step was to contact the doctor, which we did. He confirmed my diagnosis and prescribed an antibiotic and hot compresses.

Continuing to breastfeed was fine, as Addie probably already had the germs. Within twelve hours, I was feeling better, and within twenty-four hours, I was almost back to normal. From the myriad of causes listed (allowing your breasts to become too full, improper positioning of the baby, inadequate washing of hands, not getting enough rest), one can only conclude they really don't know what specifically causes the problem. Nevin is convinced that it was lack of rest. Every day I promise that I will take a nap, but something always captures my attention and I forget. I guess the infection will teach me. Nature has a way of letting you know.

Because Adelyn handled her DPT shot so well, the doctor suggested another pneumogram to retest her heart rate and respiration trends. It's the first step toward removing the machine. Addie must have two consecutive good pneumograms to consider her system stable enough to function without a machine.

I called our monitor company representative to set up an appointment, and they made two housecalls to complete the test. Addie's monitor was connected to a recorder, her breathing and respiration were recorded for twelve hours, and the results were sent to our neonatologist. We must also keep a log of her awake times since they produce different readings. The doctor is only interested in sleeping-readings. We are anxiously awaiting the results.

Tricia, a friend of mine, called the other day. Her baby is one month old, and her voice had that familiar strained quality. "I have to get out," she said, "Let's get together. " I remember that only one month ago I had said similar words to my mother, and she had come to my rescue. The first trip out is the hardest because you no longer simply grab your keys and your purse and remember to lock the door behind you. There are now new motions to go through, and you're afraid to take the first tentative steps on your own. Pack the diaper bag. (What do you need?) Learn how to work the stroller. (I practiced until I was proficient.) Dress the child appropriately. (How is that? You must also consider where you are going.) Calculate feeding times beforehand. Make sure you use the car seat correctly. Calculate how much time you need to do all of this. And, last of all, make sure you remember the baby! (And don't lock him or her in the car like I did recently. I ended up having to call the police, but they were very understanding.) It's now routine, but I remember when it was not. My mother took me to the local mall, which is where Tricia and I went, and I'm grateful to my mother for giving me confidence when I needed it.

Tricia and I had a good time. We traded tips, stories, and babies. Our talks during pregnancy had been helpful, but our discussions now were much more valuable. We were new mothers learning the lay of the land. Everyone else already seemed to know what we didn't. We felt stupid. It was reassuring to feel stupid together. Someday soon we would know too.

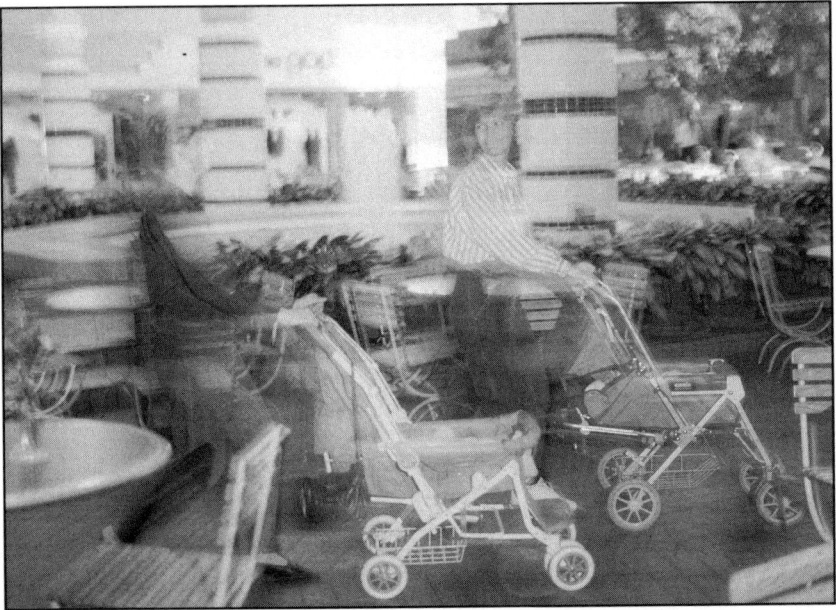

Ann and her friend, Tricia, visiting the mall with the kids. It's helpful to have a friend going through childrearing at the same time.

Trips during the day are a new learning experience. When I worked in an office, I lost touch with the rest of the world. I was always curious about what other people did with their day. Now I know. They visit the mall. The malls are filled with mothers and children, especially on rainy or otherwise unpleasant days. It's the perfect atmosphere for dealing with active children or fussy babies, and it gives mothers who haven't seen an adult all day a chance to communicate with their peers. Mothers (and some fathers) stroll from store to store or just window shop, occupying themselves and distracting their children. It's exercise for all. Everyone looks at everyone else's children. "How cute." "How old?" "I remember when mine was that little." You especially see mothers at elevators. Groups of ten get off chatting companionably, and ten more get on, nodding amiably to the group they passed. When Addie is fussy during the day, I pack her into the car and off we stroll. It's a nice outlet for both of us.

We made our first trip to the grocery store the other day. I knew eventually Nevin would not be available when we needed food. I was nervous. Addie's neck is stronger, and I can hold her to my shoulder, but it's not strong enough for her to sit in the seat of a grocery cart. How would I handle her and the cart?

For the first trip, I decided to purchase only necessary items. I had Addie at my shoulder and pushed the cart with one hand. (I am learning to do a lot of things with one hand.) As we went through the store, I noticed how others handled the same task. Baby in car seat laying across the cart. Baby in car seat in the cart. Baby wrapped in blankets at the bottom of the cart. Baby in the cart and mother pushing another cart while pulling baby along in the first.

When we got to the checkout line, Adelyn was a hit. In fact, the older gentleman behind me was so enamored of her that he emptied my cart while a young man in front of me helped him. (Chivalry is not dead!) The cashier was also delighted. She had me showing Addie to all of the other cashiers, and she was very helpful in bagging the groceries and placing them in the cart. The older gentleman asked if I could manage. I could.

I feel guilty about being so dependent on others, but I think I will just sit back and enjoy it for now. It won't last long. Addie will never be three months old again.

Dad's Thoughts

The changes in Addie are coming quickly now. Almost every day there is something new. She is developing almost faster than Annie and I can keep up. I never thought infants were very interesting, but seeing her every day and observing her at close range, I realize I have never seen the subtlety of a child's development. I am fascinated. Of course, the fact that Addie is my child does not affect my objectivity in the least. (Yeah, sure.)

The greatest of all of these recent changes are those smiles. Addie looks right at us—and grins. A lively, joyful smile. It's ample reward for any number of sleepless nights. As she gets older, I will have to be very careful about those smiles, or when she asks for a sports car at age ten, I'll go out and buy one for her.

Her smiles are the most obvious and rewarding development for us, her parents. But of far greater importance are those more subtle changes. Her increased attention span, the ability to hold her head up, and her generally growing interest in the world around her. Her increased awareness of her environment indicates cognitive development. Addie's parents, unbiased as they are, are sure this is a sign of keen intelligence. Addie takes great delight in bright or "high contrast" toys, that is, toys with both dark and light (or white) colors, not pastels. A black and white panda bear is one of her favorites. This heightened visual awareness allows Addie to more readily follow the voices, and even the footsteps, of others. Humans receive a disproportionate amount of information through their eyes, as opposed to the other four senses. It has been estimated that as much as 80 percent of the data relayed to the brain comes in through the eyes. Therefore, her development in this area is extremely important. Addie's eyes are, after all, her windows to the world.

As you may have already noticed, even Adelyn's smallest changes are of unparalleled fascination to us. In the past

few months, we have practically been able to see her growing. It seems as though she has been with us much, much
longer than three months—no, not because these have been
trying times, but because we cannot now imagine life without her. It feels like she has been with us always. Our life before Adelyn, whatever it was, is but a dim and receding
memory.

We have been aided in that perception by the elevation
of certain tasks to "routine" status. Those movements that
had seemed so alien and forced just twelve short weeks ago,
are now controlled by that part of the brain that governs our
breathing and blinking.

Holding her, changing her, rolling her into the "colic"
hold are maneuvers that can now be performed while talking on the phone, feeding the dogs, or even typing this man-
uscript. Even outings—rather, their preparation—have
become almost as much a part of everyday life as eating and
sleeping. Simply put, we are more comfortable, more confident with her than we were in the beginning. I must confess
openly, however, that Annie possesses much greater speed
and agility in handling Addie than I do.

Which brings me, however awkwardly, to another nota-
ble transition of this past month—the return of my wife. It
sounds odd to say that, I know, but you must realize that
Annie and Addie have been inseparable since Addie was
born. So the occasion of our first night out together—as a
duet rather than a trio—was for me very much like the return of a long-wandering old friend. And this was the direct
result of our becoming more confident with Addie. We no
longer felt anchored to her by the mistaken belief that we
were the only ones who could care for her.

Of course, that was not the only reason we left Addie
with Ann's parents that night. We needed to get out. It was
as simple as that. A night out with adult friends gives parents a little needed distance, a little different perspective,
and a little peace and quiet. We really don't need it often,
but when we do, we'll take it—no hesitation, no guilt, and
no calls home to the sitter (well, maybe just one).

Third Month—Pediatric Commentary by Dr. Marie Keith

Just about everything parents experience during their baby's first year is a learning experience, sometimes an anxiety-provoking one, for everyone. The baby's first shot is a good example. Most parents are apprehensive. I try to prepare my patients by discussing immunizations at the very first visit, although none are given then. Honest information helps parents deal with the baby's pain and whatever else follows—fussiness, crying, crankiness and fever. It seems all the Kishbaughs weathered this first trauma.

But Ann sounded disappointed when she had to tell her pediatrician Adelyn wasn't smiling—at least not as much as he seemed to expect. Perhaps that's where Addie's prematurity comes in. We use well-constructed scales to assess a baby's development. When a baby is premature, we have to make allowances for that baby's slow start. So Addie's smiling was a bit off schedule. But she came through with flying colors shortly thereafter.

First-time parents often tend to hover over their baby, thinking they must provide continuous amusement. But leaving a baby to entertain herself, to use her senses to find ways to comfort herself, is important, as is establishing a routine. Lots of parents don't understand the importance of following a normal pat-

tern of sleeping, eating and bodily functions, but they do help everyone out.

Parents also must learn to pick up a new baby's subtle cues about her needs and desires. This aspect of infant development and parental response is critical. It lays the groundwork for a developing flow of communication and understanding between parent and child that can last a lifetime. When Addie wailed from her stroller while in a store and Ann maneuvered groceries and child in order to hold Addie and comfort her, everyone was happier. The mother-daughter bond was strengthened and Ann's confidence grew.

Confidence increases quickly during the first few months. Despite her own newness at mothering, Ann felt able to offer comfort and advice when she joined her friend Tricia and Tricia's one-month-old daughter for a trip to the mall and some mother-to-mother chatting. Sharing like this is a great way for new mothers to increase their feelings of competence and confidence.

Ann and Nevin also are learning to integrate Addie into the life they lead, which is essential not only to development of parenting skills but also to healthy formation of the new family. Initially Addie was the center of her parent's attention and everything in the house revolved around her and her needs. Now Addie is becoming part of the family and sharing in family activities. At the same time, Ann and Nevin have learned how necessary—and rewarding—it is for them to find time for themselves and for each other. This gives a couple the balance needed for healthy parental development.

You can never really comprehend or learn all these things until you become a parent. I think Nevin was very perceptive in his comments, especially when he said: "I never thought infants were very interesting, but seeing her every day and observing her at close range, I realize that I have never seen the subtlety of a child's development." It is fascinating, which makes being a parent, not to mention being a pediatrician, one of the best things life can offer.

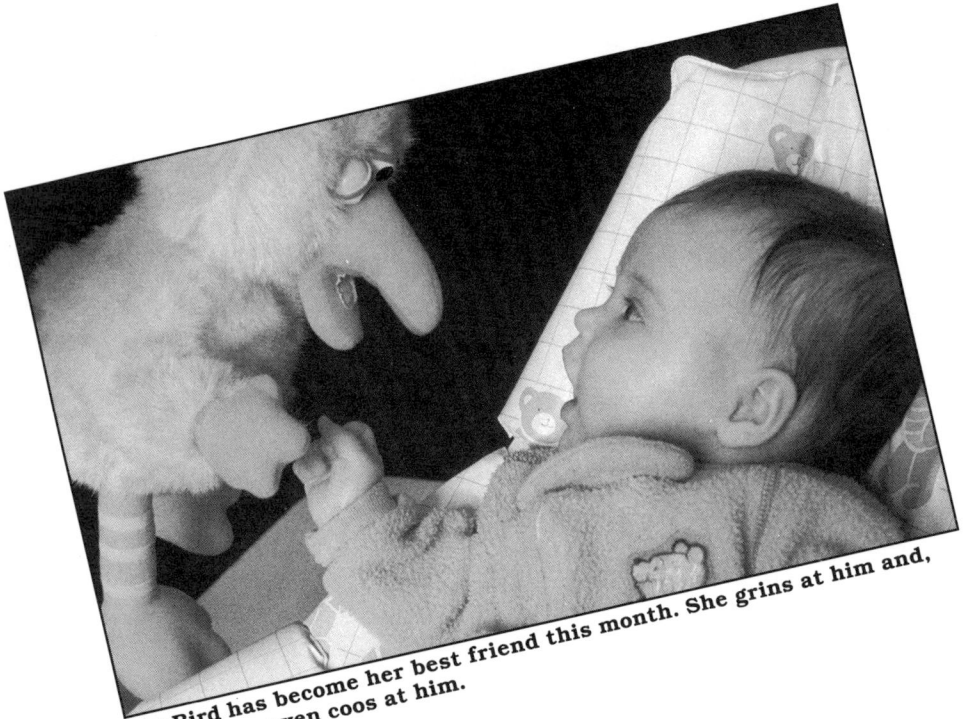
Big Bird has become her best friend this month. She grins at him and, sometimes, even coos at him.

Fourth Month

Mom's Thoughts

A significant event occurred just as Adelyn entered her fourth month: she give up her late night feeding. It happened suddenly. She just didn't wake up one night...or the next...or the next. In fact, Addie went overboard, sleeping twelve hours straight and skipping not one, not two, but three feedings out of six.

Was I in pain! I would awake in the morning with hard, tender breasts and breast milk all over my pajamas and the sheets. On entering her room to see if Addie was at all ready to eat, I'd find her cooing away at her crib toys and playing happily. Since I've read that I shouldn't disturb this crucial morning play, I would wander the house waiting impatiently for a cry. At the first yelp, I would be by her cribside studying her for signs of hunger.

Amazingly, my breasts adjusted to this bizarre schedule, and just when I no longer awoke in pain, Addie decided to eat ravenously throughout the day. Now I didn't have enough milk. We supplemented her with some formula (It's not nice to fool with Mother Nature, Addie!) until she had finally decided what her needs were. Addie settled on four meals throughout the day, with the last one taken in early evening. She still sleeps twelve hours at night, but now she remembers to eat enough during the day.

I realize that most mothers would love a schedule like this, but I miss our nighttime feedings. It was our special time. We would cuddle to the sound of the ticking clock. I feel like it's her first day of school, my first letting go. Pleasant dreams, Addie Ruth. I'm here if you need me.

Addie loves her morning play. She awakens slowly and begins cooing to various objects placed within her gaze. Since she likes to sleep on her back, she is easily amused. Addie is quite content for an hour or more to look around examining her toys, the shadows on the wall, the mobile above her bed, and, her latest discovery—her hands. She has not yet figured out that they belong to her, and at this time, they're fun for her to watch as they dance in and out of her line of vision. Everything is new and wonderful. If only we could bottle such feelings.

A more significant event for Addie was the discovery of her thumb. She's been looking for it since day one, and while she occasionally found it, it was only by accident, and she couldn't repeat it. Now Addie can find her thumb at will. It gives her great comfort and solace when she needs it and when I'm not as readily available as she might wish.

It's wonderful to watch her capture her thumb as it is a great tribute to her increasingly adept hand/eye coordina-

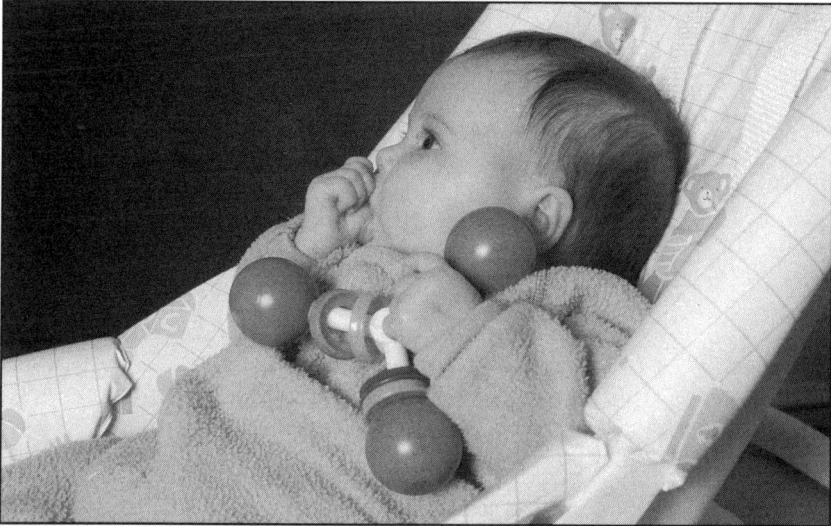

Addie found her thumb one day and has been sucking on it ever since.

tion. She slides her open hand down her face so that eyes and nose are covered momentarily. The thumb then grazes her mouth as the hand is swept down, and on feeling this, she pops it in. (As the month has progressed, she has learned to bring it to her mouth more readily when she isn't tired.) It sticks out awkwardly as she hasn't learned that her thumb bends, but it is really cute. Loud sucking now resounds through the house as it is transmitted through the intercom. Many times I know to ready myself as she'll soon discover that her thumb is not quite what she wants. One of the most beautiful sights is to see her lying in her crib on her back, one hand with thumb in her mouth and the other outstreched with open palm, and her head pressed against her black-and-white panda. She has found security in our world.

It's been gratifying and so much fun to watch Addie reach out more to the world. She strains to touch the baby in the mirror (very shyly, I might add). She jerkily raises her arm to jangle the crib gym and swipes repeatedly when her hand successfully reaches its destination. (The legs kick

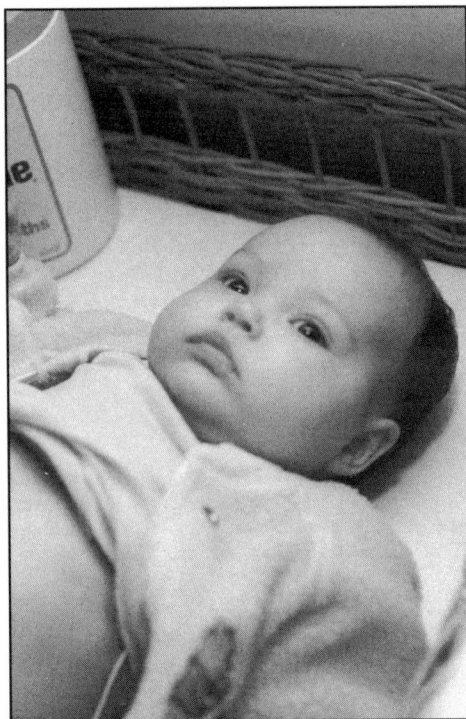

Adelyn on her changing table. Note the electrode wire that connects her to the apnea monitor.

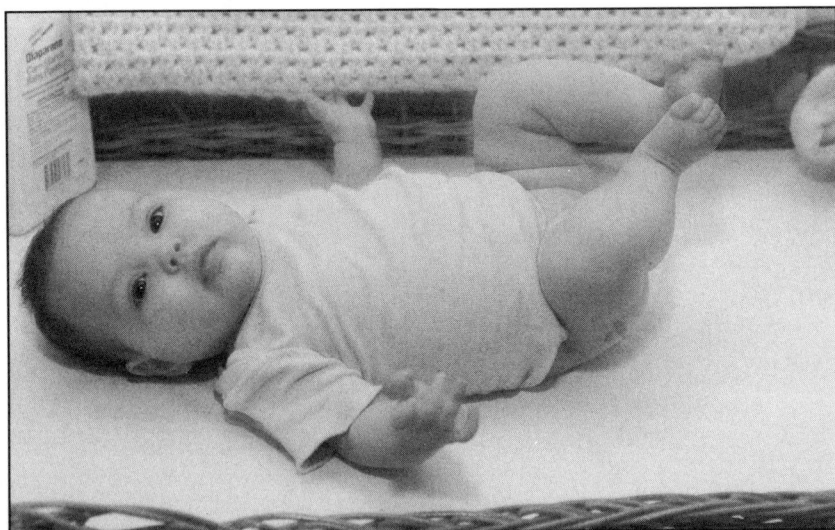

Adelyn likes to kick her legs in the air on the changing table. She is learning to control her limbs—and it's good exercise, too.

wildly as if it is hard to contain her joy.) As the month has progressed, she grabs the handles with certainty. She bangs herself in the eye with the rattle when trying to locate her mouth. She reaches up to gently touch my face when I stick out my tongue and seems surprised by the tongue's texture.

You can almost see the wheels turning as her eyes literally gleam as they spy their target. While her swipes were fairly wild at the beginning of the month, almost daily you can see improvement in her coordination. Toward the end of this month, when I hold an object up to her, she brings both hands from her sides as if she is going to embrace it. She'll then grab the toy with two hands and pull it in toward her mouth. She'll practice this "gathering in" until she is successful, but she frequently gets what she wants the first time. I am amazed at this development and could spend all day playing with her, but she tires easily and is soon ready for a nap after an hour of play. When her thumb goes in her mouth, I know to leave her alone.

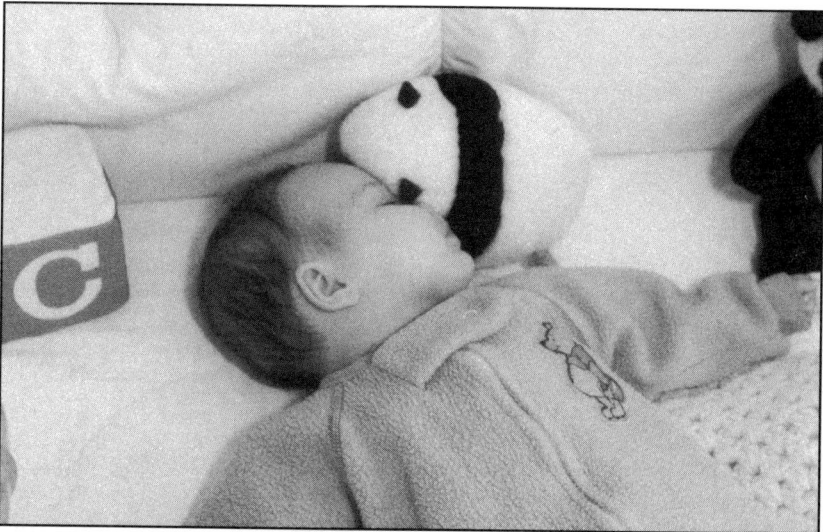

Addie likes the secure feeling of cuddling up to a favorite stuffed toy when she sleeps.

Lately, Addie has taken to staring at me and searching my face for reassurance. When we're out, I catch her staring at me as I'm doing whatever task is at hand. She watches me silently and with such intensity; however, I need only say a few words or chuck her under the chin to get a smile. In addition, I removed the infant carrier from her tub so she can kick with more abandon. Addie is a bit uncertain about this change, but she does like the fact that she can kick more freely and send the toy fish slapping against the sides. She stares constantly at me as if searching for my reactions to this activity. I keep a lively banter going and smile all the while, which isn't easy when you're trying to balance a slippery child on your wrist and concentrating on cleaning all of the little parts while searching for a good song to sing (one for which you know all the lyrics). Her watchful eyes make me feel so important.

As the month has progressed, other changes in Addie's vision have become apparent. She will watch Nevin and me leave a room, her eyes and head following our course. While I noticed last month that she was attracted to red objects, it is obvious this month that yellow is the color of choice. She finally noticed Big Bird on her Sesame Street gym. She wouldn't give him the time of day before but she's crazy about him now. Addie shyly grins and sometimes even coos at him. I understand that green colors will be next followed by blue. Perhaps soon she will give Cookie Monster some needed attention.

Recently, I got the sense that her vision had changed significantly. She stares at hanging plants several feet away and loves ceiling fans that are in adjoining rooms. While Nevin and I have been her main objects of interest for a few months, she is now straining to look beyond us. The books say that she can now see as well as Nevin and I do.

With this change in her vision and her disposition, I now find that we can interest her in simple preschool books. Books with babies and picture books with nursery rhymes seem to capture her attention. Since we are very interested in promoting reading, we have established a bedtime routine that includes reading to her for as long as she will allow it, which varies depending on her mood, from five minutes to twenty minutes. Before her morning nap is also a good time.

I am becoming a regular Luciano Pavarotti. I have been singing my little heart out since the day she was born because you can only find so much to talk about when you are carrying on a one-way conversation. I am dredging up songs that I have not thought about or sung in years. It's amazing how many songs I know—not very well, but with enough lyrics to fudge it. Addie seems to like it. She stares at me and kicks her legs at my breast when she is in an active mood. It's nice to have such a receptive audience.

I recently bought a lullaby tape as I found that, besides "Kumbaya," I really didn't know any lullabies, and you can only sing that one for so long. Addie enjoys the soothing sound, and when she is just about to doze off but having problems, the lullaby tape sends her on her way so very peacefully. It is so rewarding to be able to do this for her. I wish I had started to learn lullabies while I was pregnant as they might have been useful during the infancy stage.

Addie is trying in her own way to communicate with us. Her babbling has increased over the months, and it is now apparent that she is experimenting with different sounds. It even seems that she may be mimicking our tones and inflections. If I speak softly, she babbles quitely. As I get louder, her tones become bolder. Addie is most talkative on her changing table. We can keep a dialogue going for about ten to fifteen minutes. First I will talk, stop, and look at her expectantly. She will then try to find her voice. It takes her a few minutes and sounds quite rusty at first. If I talk again and wait, she will eventually give another croak. As this continues, she warms up to the exercise and sounds come forth more readily and more excitedly. Addie is entranced by whispering, and coos softly in reply while giving me a shy smile. Loud tones scare her (she actually jumps with eyes wide), so I try to talk in a low and slow voice.

Addie is very vocal when she is not happy about something. We call it her complaining voice. A few times at night, we have been awakened by her "shouting." (There is no other word for it. It is not crying but very loud and angry tones that continue for as long as ten minutes or more.) The first time I heard it, I thought she was experimenting with a new voice so I let her continue for a bit. On finally entering her room, I discovered that she had wiggled out of her covers, and I can only conclude that she must have been cold. She went back to sleep easily.

I have finally learned something about Addie that should be helpful as the year progresses. She is a quiet baby and is startled and upset easily by great outbursts. When I am in a bouncy mood and exhibit louder behavior than usual, she seems very startled at my actions and may even cry. I have to quiet myself down for her so as not to scare her. My books suggest that you adapt your personality to the child. I am learning to handle her gently and soothingly. I just get so darned excited sometimes!

Dad's Thoughts

Annie and Addie are becoming quite a pair. What I mean is that they are becoming quite interdependent. Addie is a *baby* now as opposed to an *infant*. We considered her infancy over at about three months when she developed cheeks and round fingers and began to realize who we were. An arbitrary distinction to be sure, but it helps categorize her development.

I tell you this only to clarify the statement that since Addie has become a baby, she has become more attached to Ann and less so to me. During infancy, Annie and I were almost interchangeable to her. She would direct her focus on whomever was with her. Now, however, Addie's eyes will follow her mother out of the room, and she will gaze randomly about until Annie returns—never mind that I am talking to her or rocking her.

This attachment, of course, is natural—and understandable. Annie is the primary parent, feeding her, chang-

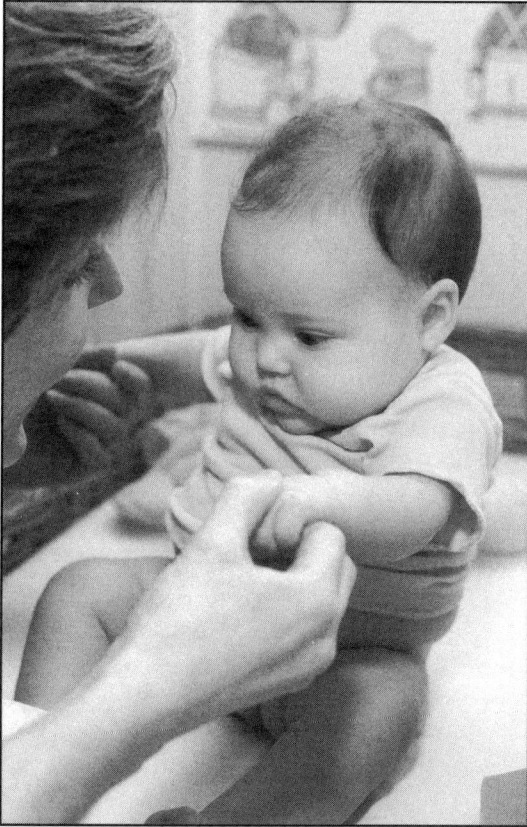

**Annie pulls Addie up to a sitting position—
just to give her a little practice.**

ing her, playing with her all day. Such symbiosis rarely
leaves room for a third party.

Also, I have not been around much lately. My time has
been occupied with a project out of town, and I have been
spending a lot of hours in the darkroom at night. With all
factors considered, there is little time for the proverbial
father/daughter bonding. It is not that she does not respond
to me, she just does not respond the way she does to Ann.
As I said before, it is completely natural and understandable—I just don't particularly like it.

Perhaps this is why I find myself looking forward more
and more to the years ahead when Addie is walking and

talking. I realize that I'm getting a little ahead of myself here; after all, she is still only four months old. But when she reaches the toddler/young child stage, Annie and I will be more equal parents. I hope so, anyway.

Perhaps this is why I find myself watching young children in supermarkets and other places more intently now. I am genuinely fascinated by them. Little kids, like dogs, are inherently funny. They are innocent, observant, and painfully honest. My brother, Eric, often watches his girlfriend's little girl. Desiree is six years old and quite fond of Eric. Yet she realizes, clearly, that my brother is not a parent. "Eric," she will say, "you don't know the first thing about kids." Pretty sharp, don't you think?

When I was that age, I was a bit less judgmental. My mother used to love to tell the story of the day I came into the kitchen, tugged on her skirt hem, and asked, quite innocently, "Mom, were there trees in your day?" She did not find the incident amusing until some years later.

So, strange as it may seem, I am looking forward to the time when Addie Ruth will point out my obvious flaws. I only hope that I take them as good-naturedly as my brother does.

Because I have been away so much lately, Adelyn's progress seems much more dramatic to me. She is now entertained less by us than by distant objects. Her eyes are drawing in things that they could not before, and the shapes and colors mesmerize her. While it bothers us a little to be ignored by our own daughter, we realize how exciting her new world must be.

She has even begun to notice our two dogs, who constantly interject themselves between Addie and me. Like most people, when I talk to my child, my voice gets higher in pitch. The dogs, having grown accustomed to this voice being directed toward them all of these years, are a bit jealous. Adelyn looks at them inquisitively, but does not seem to mind the intrusion—even when they nudge her with their cold noses.

The other day, Annie suggested that I join bath time as it was beginning to be a very different experience. Remembering the last time, I was not looking forward to Addie's violent screams of protest. It is disconcerting, to say the least, to hear your child be "tortured" so. And that is really what it sounded like.

Boy was I surprised! She loved it. She kicked and splashed and flung her arms about, sometimes pushing off of the small tub with her legs with such force that she would have banged her head on the other end if it were not for Annie's quick gestures.

Addie is getting very strong. I can see already that by the time she is walking, she will be hard to hold down. Even on the changing table, she flails her legs wildly, pushing off any solid surface. Her motor skills are developing nicely. With so many changes occurring in this one month, we can not wait to see what next month brings.

Postscript: Addie Ruth's pneumogram was normal. She will be tested again in four weeks.

Fourth Month—Pediatric Commentary by Dr. Marie Keith

When an infant reaches the three- to four-month stage, some exciting milestones are achieved that are a delight for parents to behold. As Ann and Nevin's story this month illustrates, the learning of new behavior is a beautiful process to observe. The uninitiated observer may miss the subtleties or find the unrefined movement or sound to be without meaning.

Up until now, the newborn has made good use of all of its senses—vision, hearing, taste, smell and touch—to perceive its world. The innate reflexes of rooting and sucking have helped the baby find nourishment, the startle reflex allows response to unexpected movement or sound, and the grasp reflex lets a baby cling briefly to an object at hand. The newborn also has muscle strength and tone that provide movement of the arms and legs and the ability to lift the head up for short periods.

By three months, the baby has had some ninety days of life experience. Much of the early days were spent adjusting to the processes of eating, waking and sleeping, and elimination. It may not always occur to us, but these routine functions of daily life are all new to the infant, and it takes practice until the infant settles into a comfortable pattern. This accomplished, the baby can now make some progress in some other spheres of activity.

Infants learn in a world without words—theirs is a preverbal understanding of the world as presented to them by their sensory input. They combine this with a trial and error approach to muscle movement and coordination, and by about three months of age, what emerges is one of the earliest manifestations of learned behavior—hand/eye coordination.

An explanation of the steps involved gives us a full appreciation of what the baby has learned. Imagine first that your head rested on a pillow and you were unable to pick it up; your eyes mostly gazed straight ahead and could focus best on what was about twelve to eighteen inches away, and you kept your arms predominantly to the side of your head or your body. It could be difficult to conceive of hand/eye coordination developing in this state, yet this is where an infant begins. Then the baby develops coordination by using the increasing acuity of the senses, the increased muscle tone that supports the head, and repetitive trial and error movement of its arms so that she can flex and rotate her muscles to bring her hands into midline view.

The newborn infant lying on her tummy or on the parent's shoulder can lift her head briefly to look about, but as her neck muscles tire, the head comes crashing down on the mattress or shoulder. A newborn lying on her back is unable to pick up her head at all, and when held in a semi-upright or sitting position, the head must be supported or it flops backward. By three months of age, through exercise and practice, infants have the muscle strength and tone to hold their heads up for relatively long periods without tiring, and also can bend and turn them.

On a parallel course of development, again through exercise and practice, the infant has managed to move her arms in such a way that they begin to move over the trunk of the body and the face instead of being predominantly at the side. Thus the infant begins to suck her thumb, inadvertently grasp her own hair or ears, scratch her cheeks, and look at her hands. The baby does all this as movement of her arms to the midline is being mastered.

On yet another avenue of development, the newborn's eyesight gradually changes. At birth an infant will gaze strongly at a significant stimulus, such as a face or an object with high contrast colors presented within a foot or two of her eyes. The new baby will gaze intently at light and seems to appreciate form and movement although the baby "sees" indistinctly. Tracking or following movement over a short distance occurs. In the interval between one and two months, it becomes obvious to the observer that the baby will visualize and track objects that are perhaps six to eight feet away, or farther. When shifting gaze from far to near, the infant often crosses her eyes as she attempts to adjust her focus.

Now that the baby has some control of the neck muscles, advancing visual abilities, and the newfound skills of moving the hands to a place in front of her face, the next steps fall neatly into place. The infant visualizes an object and also sees her hand in front of her face. The strength of the neck and tracking with the eyes allow the baby to follow the movement of her hands which at first seem to be some-what random or flailing, but then become quite directed toward the object that is seen. At this moment, the infant has learned, in its most rudimentary state, the process of hand/eye coordination. In a very gradual manner, she begins to know that she can direct her hands toward an object in her sight.

At this point, basic infant toys such as a light-weight rattle or a colorful mobile begin to have some meaning for the baby. Parents can participate in the infant's learning process by offering these toys for stimulation at times when the baby is quiet and receptive. It is a joyful moment for both parent and baby as the baby learns she can direct the movement of her hands and the process of hand/eye coordination unfolds.

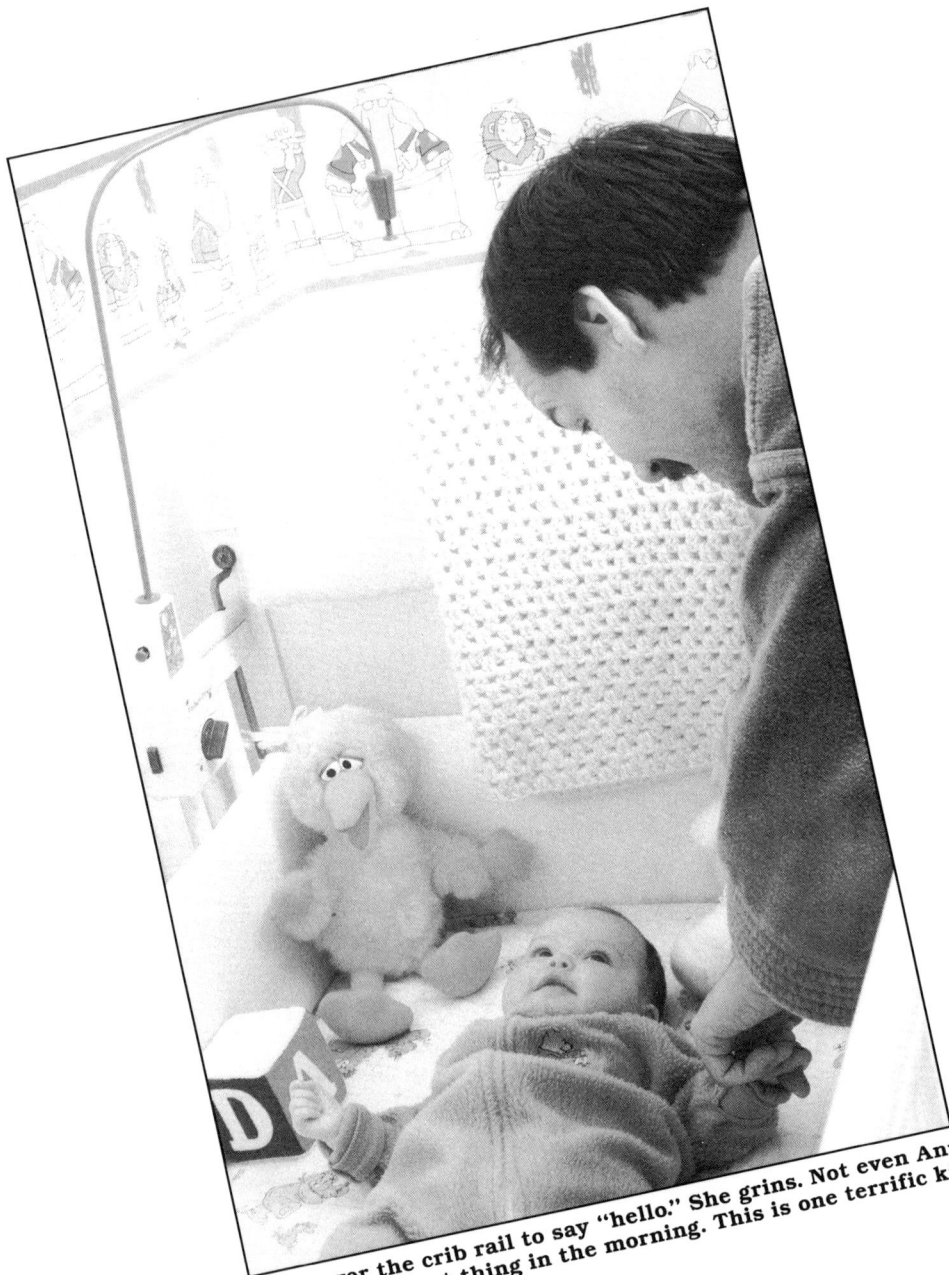

I peer over the crib rail to say "hello." She grins. Not even Ann smiles at me first thing in the morning. This is one terrific kid I've got.

Fifth Month

Mom's Thoughts

Addie began her fifth month at the doctor's office for her four-month check-up. This visit was a bit different—Addie screamed and howled at the strange faces attending her and the hands gently prodding her. Tears poured down her cheeks. Poor baby. On the positive side, she liked the oral polio vaccine this time, but the DPT shot had the same effect. It was a fairly traumatic time, but Addie again fell into a deep sleep as soon as it was over.

Her weight was average, but alas, she may be destined to be a midget. With parents who are on the short side, I'm not really surprised; however, I am less upset because I remember my sister Ruth's experience. Eight years ago when her daughter, Amy Ruth (Ruth is a very special name in our family, too), was Addie's age, she called my mother in a panic. "Amy is going to be a shrimp," she exclaimed tearfully. Amy Ruth is now the tallest girl in her class.

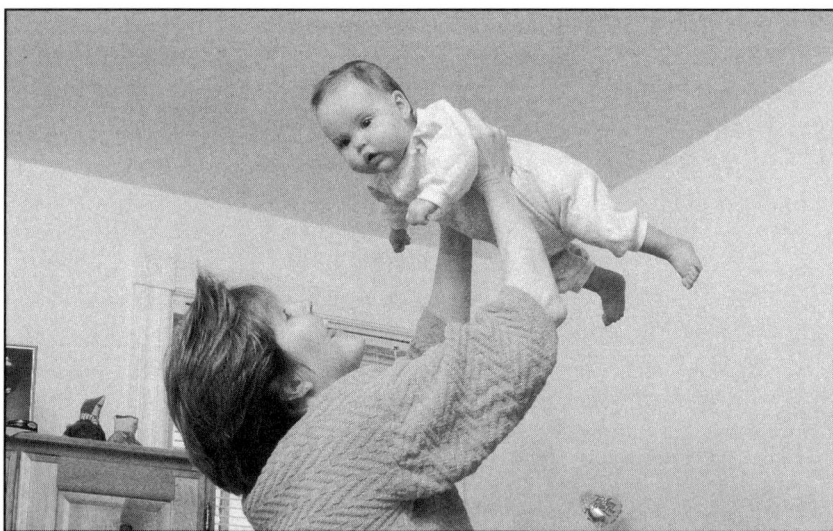

Addie is not quite sure if she likes this particular view of the world.

This time I came to the doctor's office armed with a written list of questions and as soon as the doctor finished Addie's physical exam, I pulled out my list. "Addie doesn't like to lie on her stomach," I explained. "Will this be a problem or retard her development? Should I place her on her stomach more often?" He replied that it would not be a problem for her development, but he would like to see her spend part of the day in other positions so she doesn't develop a flat head. Addie does have quite a bald spot on the back of her head where she has rubbed off the hair by moving her head from side to side, but her head is shaped beautifully—at least now.

I was also a bit concerned because she has had such a hard time leaving my breasts after she is finished eating. Addie will complain loudly when I finally stop her at the late-day feedings after twenty minutes at each breast. I believe she would continue all evening if I didn't stop her. She also associates me with milk all of the time, and it's hard for me to hold her and play with her because of this. The doctor explained that this would lessen with time. Her whole life now is still sleeping and eating, for the most part.

We discussed starting solids, and he explained his flexibility on this issue. Sometime between four and six months, solids should be started very slowly with cereal or fruits (except citrus) as starter foods. He explained how to put the spoon in her mouth and suggested that I begin early in the day. He stressed beginning solids when I felt comfortable with it and when Adelyn seems to be demanding more. Since my sister had commented that her son, now two years old, had such a hard time handling solids, I'm in no big hurry. I'll take my cue from Addie Ruth.

I also mentioned that Addie seemed to be smiling and babbling less than she had previously. The doctor smiled and said not to worry, it only meant that she was involved in something else for the time being. I have to keep telling myself that what Addie does is normal for Addie. I also have to remember not to take things personally, but you know how it is. Those smiles just make your day!

One of my books says that mothers may become "impatient" with children at this stage because the children are less dependent on them. Another book says that I should expect "strangeness" as a result of the mid-brain becoming developed at this age. I feel better on reading these statements because I am searching for an explanation for our being out of sync.

After Addie began smiling, I was the key to her world. She would smile readily at every little thing I said or did. It was so gratifying. She now regards me solemnly, and when I do get a smile, I have worked very hard to get it. She gets cranky or "feisty" (she rarely cries anymore) when she doesn't like something, and she has chosen not to like her bath again. I am baffled and feel that perhaps I have done something to cause these reactions but, of course, that is not rational. I realize now that this is the first stage of a very primitive form of communication between us. I am no longer a novelty, but someone with whom she needs to learn to express herself, and she is trying in her own way.

Despite Addie's somber demeanor, her biggest achievement this month was laughing out loud when I was holding her while talking on the phone with a friend. While she has made small giggles in the past, this particular laugh welled up from her belly and sounded like someone had told her the best joke. (Actually, she was looking at the ceiling fan in the next room.) She laughed. I laughed. She laughed some more, and I laughed some more. My friend on the other end of the phone laughed. We shared this laughter for at least thirty seconds. Addie and I were belly to belly. It was such a special moment. Unfortunately, I don't think Addie knows

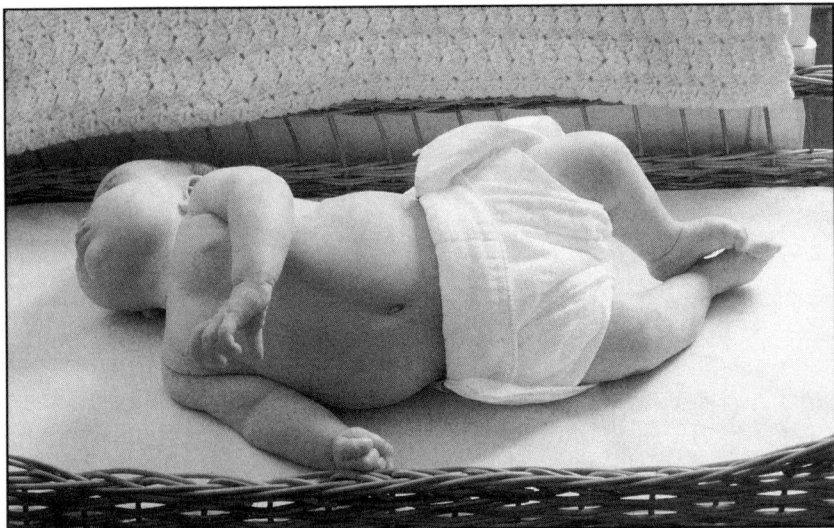

Addie's changing table "twist." It won't be long before she ends up on her belly.

how to repeat it yet. Well, Addie, it looks like you have your father's sense of humor.

Addie has not yet rolled over from her back to her stomach, and I again remind myself that what Addie does is normal for Addie. (They will not ask her in a future job interview when she first rolled over on her stomach!) She *will* walk someday—and it will be on her own schedule. (And, they won't ask her when she walked either!) There are signs that she has the capability to roll over. When she is on the changing table, she performs "the twist" and cranes her head around to look behind her, which lifts her torso toward one side. If she followed through with her legs, she would find herself on her side, but her toes are busily playing with each other as they wave high in the air above her. (Addie is very adept with her toes. This won't do her a lot of good in life, but I'm still proud of this strange accomplishment.) Because Addie hates being on her stomach, I can see that she has no real incentive to move in that direction, but perhaps someday soon it will occur to her that there are other ways of looking at the world. Addie's hand/eye coordination is becoming quite good, and she is trying to reach with one hand now although she is not that successful yet. (That is, she wasn't until this morning when she reached out grabbed my nipple *very* hard!) Everything given to her goes in her mouth, and a chain of colored rings can be played with for quite a long time because she can maneuver them easily from hand to hand. Recently, I placed a suction cupped toy on the tray of her swing (but did not activate the swing) to see what she would do. She grabbed the ears of the little bear and pulled herself upright to put it in her mouth. She was furious when it slipped from her grasp and bounced back into place. The thumb went into her mouth, and she observed the bear coldly for a few minutes. Then she tried again. And again. Sometimes she was successful and sometimes not, but she kept trying. By her vocalizing, we knew when she was not successful.

I am gratified by the moments when I have aroused her interest. I am sure other mothers must worry as I do about providing the proper stimulation. The books baffle me. Stimulate them, but don't overstimulate them. Let them discover on their own. Mother is the best plaything. When she is content to just lie in her crib examining her toys and kicking, I worry that I am not interacting enough with her. If she fusses when I attempt to play with her, I worry that I am overstimulating her and hampering her independence. (Addie, tell me what to do!) I try to go by her cues, but at times, I think she may get drowsy because of boredom. I believe this is where instincts come in. Nevin reminds me that mine are very good. Thanks, Nevin.

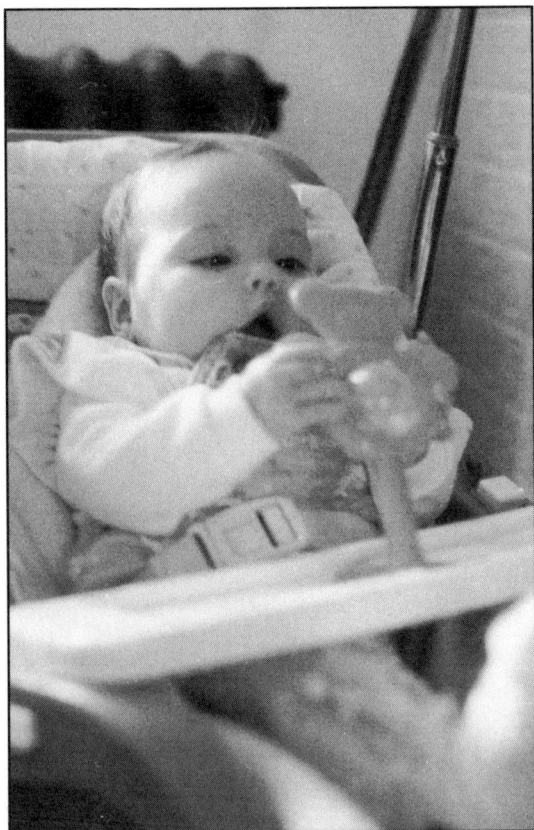

Addie tries to pull herself upright with the help of a suction-cupped toy.

While Addie stopped vocalizing for a few weeks, she returned to this activity toward the middle of this month. She began again with "raspberries," and then moved on to "ah" for a few days. "Goo" is the current favorite, and high-pitched squeals now startle the pets from their afternoon naps. Nevin swears she said "da" recently.

Addie talks a lot to Nevin. He has been home recuperating from back surgery, and it's as if Addie has discovered a new playmate. (One of the reasons Nevin had the surgery was because he couldn't hold her or pick her up.) She beams broadly when he talks to her (I'm so glad she's smiling again!) and coos in delight. It's wonderful for him since she previously seemed to ignore him for me. I think it's beginning to dawn on her that there are *two* people who are very significant in her life.

Dad's Thoughts

A few weeks can make a remarkable difference. Just when I had resigned myself to being odd man out in our family, Adelyn has decided that she is quite fond of me after all. She grins whenever I talk to her and looks for me when she hears my voice. I talk to her over Ann's shoulder while she nurses, and my little girl has, on occasion, stopped nursing to smile up at me. All of this has been quite encouraging to me, so much so that the first thing I do in the morning is look in on her. I'm usually up by 6:30 A.M., and I slip quietly into her room to see if she's awake. She usually is. Surprisingly, it will be another hour before Addie "asks" to be fed. I peer over the crib rail to say "Hello." She grins. Not even Ann smiles at me first thing in the morning. This is one terrific kid I've got.

I would like to think that Adelyn's response to me is the result of an awareness that I am her father, as important a figure as her mother. But Ann contends that it's simply because Addie thinks I'm funny looking. The truth is that Addie Ruth is becoming more social. She will sometimes smile at strangers, responding to gentle, friendly voices. We no longer worry about her being fussy when we take her somewhere, and when Ann and I wanted to go out for dinner two weeks ago, we decided to take Addie with us. Ann's mother would gladly have watched her for us, as she has done many times, but we wanted to see how we would fare on our own. Obviously, we weren't about to try a four-star restaurant, but we did want good food and a pleasant atmosphere. Ann suggested another criterion—a lively place. If Addie began to cry, Ann said, the background noise would minimize the disruption to the other patrons.

Ours was not an original idea. At the restaurant, we met another couple who had brought their little girl who was, we found out, only two weeks older than Adelyn. They had been taking their daughter along since she was a few weeks old. Unlike us, they didn't use a car seat. They simply put the baby in their laps during the meal. We asked for a table for four so that we could put Addie's car seat on the table, and other than the fact that the table was a bit crowded, the dinner went very smoothly. Adelyn slept the whole time.

This gives us an extra degree of freedom, at least while Addie is small. We did, of course, plan the evening around her schedule, leaving for dinner after her last feeding and after she had fallen asleep. While this was the first occasion we took Adelyn to a public place (other than the mall), we have always believed that Addie should be a mobile child. We hope that keeping her mobile will reduce any feelings of fear or apprehension she may have, in the future, toward strangers or unusual situations. We'll see if our theory works.

Taking Addie with us, even to her grandparents' for the evening, may soon be easier. The apnea monitor may be leaving our house. We are awaiting the results of the second, and hopefully final, pneumogram. At this point, I think our greatest hurdle is to overcome the anxiety the loss of this security system will cause. Although we dislike the intrusion of this device into our lives, we still rely on it to some extent. When the monitor is gone, it will be like flying

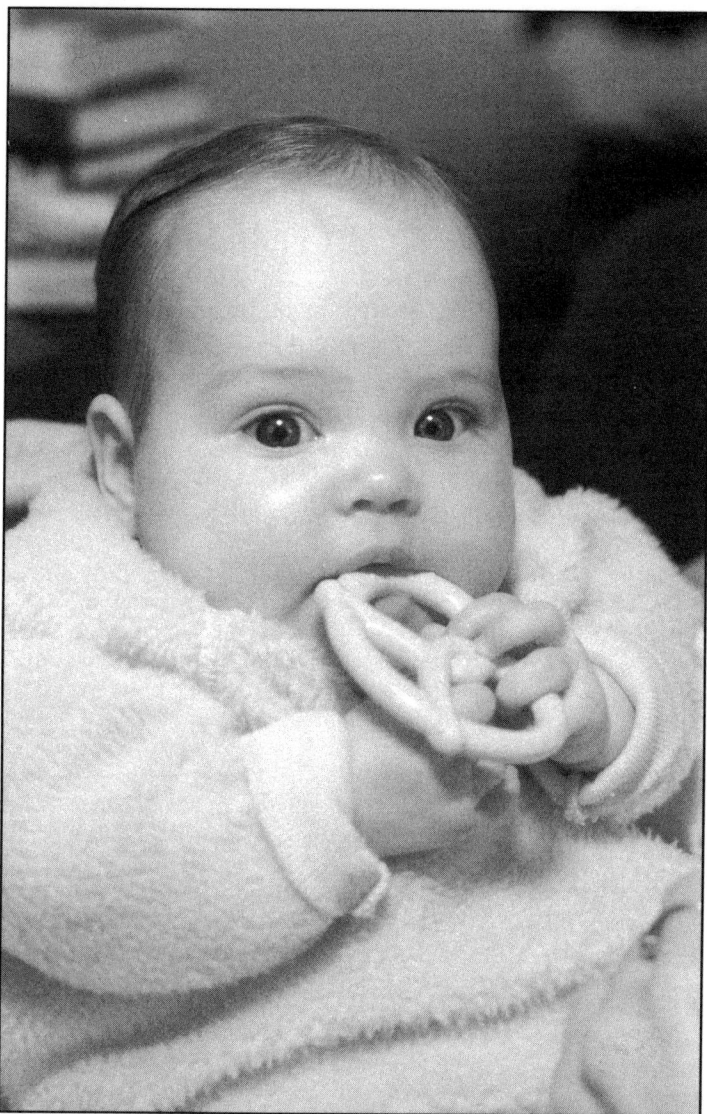

Exploration always begins with the mouth.

solo for the first time. I'm sure the first few nights will be nerve racking. We'll probably be running in to check on her every ten minutes, but I'm sure we'll regain our confidence quickly.

Fifth Month—Pediatric Commentary by Dr. Marie Keith

The wings of the butterfly slowly unfurl, flutter a few times, stretch out to their full size and suddenly a beautiful new creature emerges. Something equally wonderful happens to the young infant when she reaches roughly four to five months of age, as the social being gradually unfolds in subtle but obvious ways.

Just as the development of hand/eye coordination came about as innate reflexes were modified by trial and error, the social development of the child is built on a foundation composed of the characteristics with which the baby is born and the experiences she has from the moment of birth.

Many careful observers of infant development have theorized that the essential temperament of the child is established at birth and is already obvious in the newborn nursery. How the baby responds to stimulation, accommodates to changes, settles down after a disturbance, regulates feeding and sleeping, and establishes patterns seems to be related to the distinctive temperament with which the baby is born. So a glimpse of the personality of the child can be caught from her earliest days.

The development of a social smile, which begins at about two months, is the next stage on the path to sociability. Initially the smile is tentative and Mom or Dad may not be sure that what they are seeing is not just wishful expectation. But soon the smile becomes real and delights the hearts of parents, siblings, family, and friends. The baby has learned to show her enjoyment and comfort in a situation by gracing it with a smile. The smile becomes a very strong tool for social interaction.

During the early weeks of the infant's ability to smile, she usually is not discriminating. Any face that approaches with merely a pleasant demeanor may provoke a smile. A fanciful toy or a strange antic also might produce a smile. But then the baby's visual discrimination begins to sharpen and she begins to see faces in a new way—observing features and seeming to store the information in memory. When Ann talks about how Addie looked at her solemnly and was very hard to engage in fun, in a way she was noticing Addie at work storing information in her brain. The stored information makes it possible for the baby to recognize a familiar face or know that a face is different.

The most familiar face that baby comes to know is that of its primary caretaker, usually the mother. The mother is the baby's safe refuge and, for a while, seems to be the recipient of most of the smiles. The poor father and others who have been there all along just don't seem to get the same recognition. At this point, "stranger anxiety" begins where the baby has come to recognize the face that she knows best and regards all others as foreign.

Fortunately, there are also other mechanisms at work in the development of the child's personality and sociability so that those who appear as strangers don't remain so for long. In loving and warm interactions with the child, the other significant people in her life begin to be showered with smiles again in what has developed as the basic elements of trust. The baby has come to know that while her mother may still be the first place to seek comfort, there are

other adults with whom she can be happy and feel the radiance of love.

Coupled with this security is a new ability to produce a sound when the baby smiles—at first a very primitive sound but one that serves as the basis for happy peals of laughter. Now the baby can respond with a happy laugh to a situation that makes her feel good. In this way, a social being evolves from the basic temperament of the infant who now can interact with those around her by smiling and laughing.

At about the fifth month, mothers begin to ask me about starting their babies on solids, just as Ann was wondering this month. I'll discuss this important matter next month.

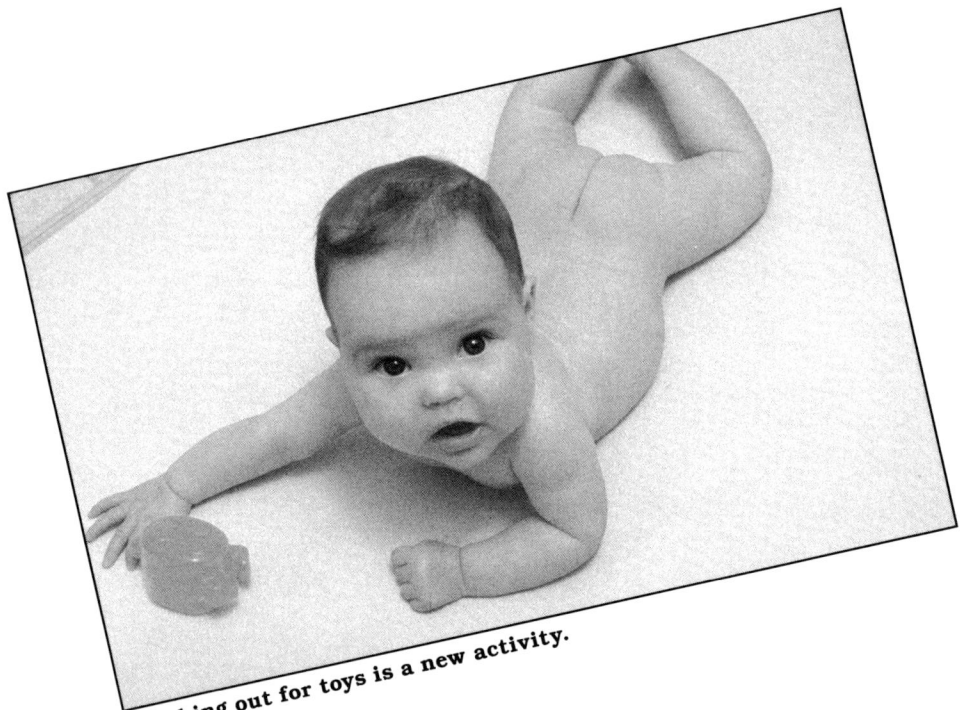

Reaching out for toys is a new activity.

Sixth Month

Mom's Thoughts

A whole new world opened up for Adelyn this month: food, glorious food. And does she love it! My first clue came when she reached out her hands one day as the bottle of fluoride vitamins (fluoride is frequently prescribed for breast-fed babies) entered her vision. When I pulled out the dropper, she grabbed my hands, navigated the dropper to her mouth, and sucked it vigorously instead of pushing it out or lolling it around in her mouth as she had done previously.

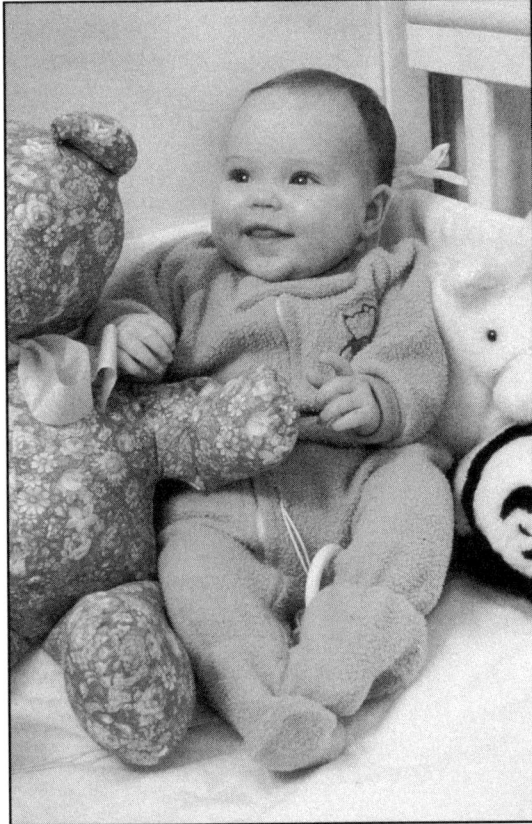

A portrait of Adelyn at six months.

Later that same day, she was sitting on my lap as I ate a banana. Her eyes were gleaming at that banana, and they followed the banana's route showing true desire. Then her hands flew out. I let her gum it a little just to get the taste, and she got very upset when I had to disengage her tiny little fingers from their grip. Hmmm, I thought, I guess she's ready. Another telltale sign was when I noticed that she kept pushing up her feeding times throughout the day as if she were not satisfied.

Our pediatrician recommended cereal or fruits for her first food, so, of course, I chose a very ripe, mashed banana. Addie was thrilled. Her mouth opened wide like a little bird, and she leaned in toward the oncoming spoon. At the same time, her hand grabbed the spoon to inspect its contents. In one sucking motion, the bananas were gone, and she was eager for more. Although I was cheerfully chatting about bananas, apes, and Tarzan, Addie was somber. This eating was serious business. When we finished her prepared portion, she wanted more.

Next came cereal, more fruits, and now she's about to try vegetables. So far we haven't tried anything Addie doesn't like to eat—or like to play with! We can't eat in front of her either. At a family dinner, she watched me intently from her perch on my lap and then had a fit when I wouldn't give her some of my dinner. Although it wasn't her regular feeding time, I opened a jar of fruit and fed her also.

On a very hot day at my sister's house, Addie again made her wishes known. She *wanted* the drink I was having, so my sister found a child's cup with a teacher beaker and gave her some diluted apple juice. Addie held it very well with two hands, and although half of it ended up all over her T-shirt and me, the other half reached its destination. (She looks so grown-up with a cup in her hands!) All of this has also led to my letting her gum an occasional zwieback. I, of course, monitor her closely when she is partaking of this treat on my lap, but she is having a lot of fun with such new "toys." She still enjoys breastfeeding, but she seems more satisfied now when she's finished, and eating solids is a fun new activity for all of us.

Addie has become much more physical in her play this month, which has led to her enjoyment of all kinds of new games. Dad throws her in the air and Addie giggles madly. "Peekaboo" and "Pattycake" are finally enjoyed. Addie giggles quietly when I reappear from behind my hands and grab her, and grins with glee as we "roll it and pat it." "This Little Piggy" is also a great favorite.

In addition, Addie found her toes one morning as she was being diapered and has been chewing them ever since at every opportunity. She looks like she is working out with Jane Fonda when she has her naked playtime before her bath. She puts her legs straight out, then raises them up,

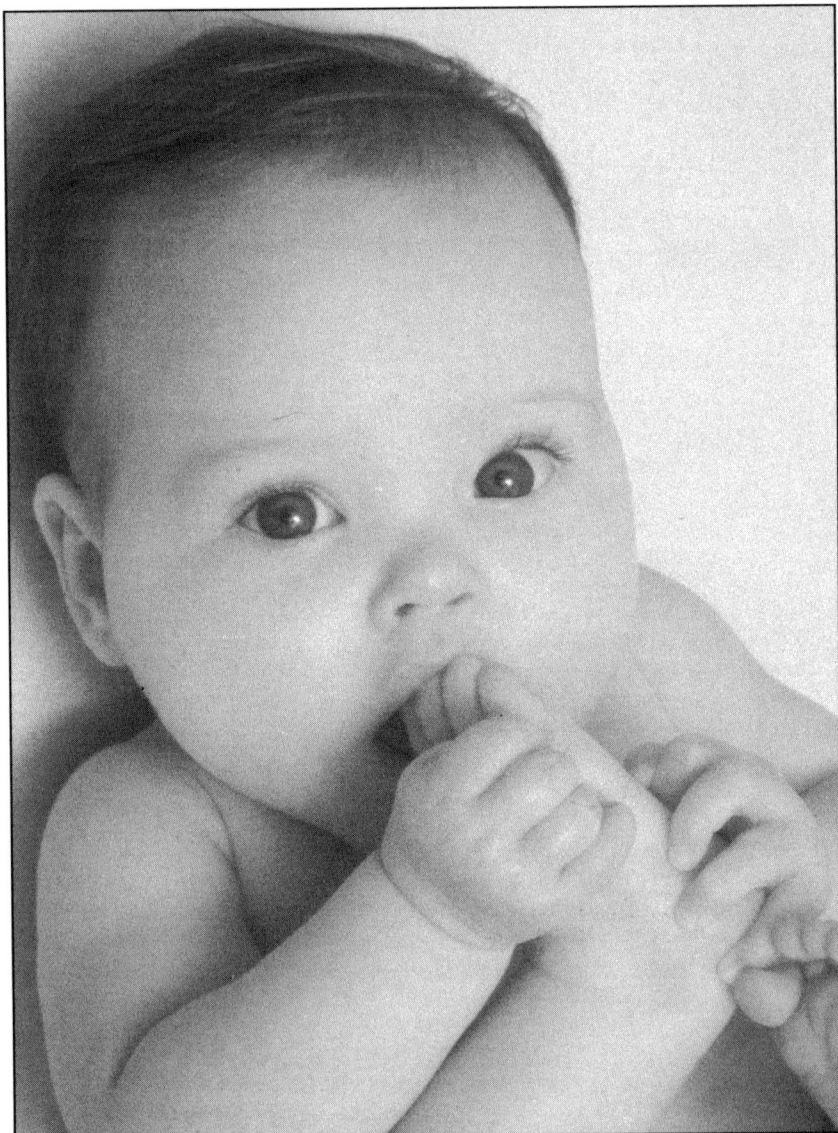

One day, Addie found her toes. I envy her flexibility.

lowers her feet down, and pulls on each foot until one responds willingly and comes toward her mouth. Chomp, chomp. Eventually, the foot pops out, and the process is repeated—over and over and over. Funny, I never tire of watching it—over and over and over.

Addie also turned over this month, which was a great milestone. Again during naked playtime, while on her stomach, her arm went straight out, and with a swift but subtle movement, she was looking at the ceiling. Addie was blase (she *has* seen the ceiling before), but I was clapping and cheering. Her greatest joy is reaching behind her on the changing table, grabbing the diaper wipe canister, and maneuvering it so it is on her stomach where she can chew on its bottom.

As demonstrated by her changing table antics, Addie has also begun to search out playthings instead of waiting to have them brought to her. It doesn't happen that often yet, but occasionally she will grab a toy on her own in the playpen or her crib. I've also seen her pick up a toy after she has dropped it. Similarly, objects in my hands or within reach are no longer safe. This became apparent when she reached out to grab a hot cup of tea I was drinking. Even though you read the warnings in books, it takes a real-life situation to bring the message home. Nobody was hurt and am I ever aware of the possibility of danger as Addie's abilities develop.

Addie cannot yet sit on her own and doesn't really like being propped up for longer than one minute, but when pulled to a sitting position, she can hold her head up well and balance for a few seconds before toppling over. I am fascinated by her hand coordination as she tries to pick up objects and bring them to her mouth. She is very creative in accomplishing anything she sets her mind to. Some actions, of course, are accidental, but others are *so* deliberate. I never appreciated my hands as much as I do now. To think that I learned as she is learning by years of trial and error. Amazing!

Babbling continues to be a favorite pastime, but with one change: The air is filled with consonants—K's, B's (a lot

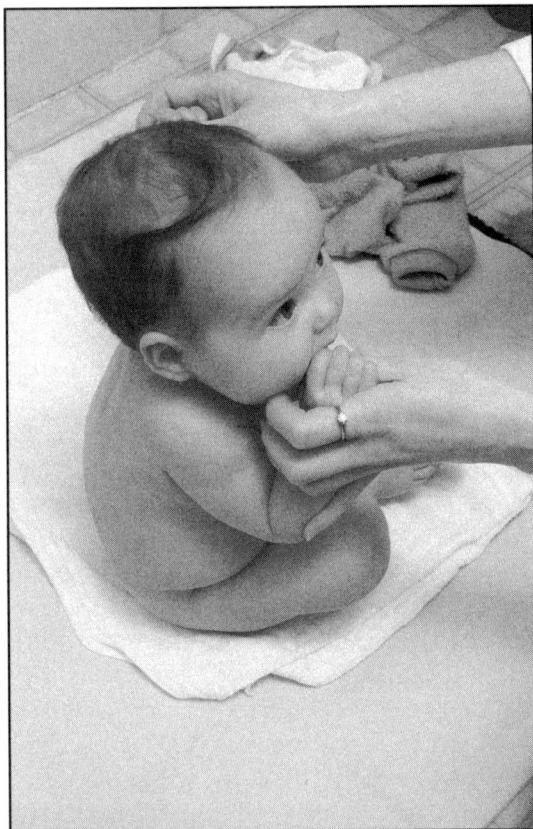

**We are encouraging her to sit up, but she's
still a little shaky yet.**

more bubbles than sound, however), and D's. We love to listen to her. I now feel like I am taking a different person with
me when we go out. In stores, she will babble away to no
one in particular when she is in the mood to be noisy. At
other times, she just wants to silently inspect each of the
packages given to her. At the grocery store, a bag of pretzels
keeps her occupied for a couple of aisles until she decides
that she would rather talk than listen. Her senses are really
getting a workout this month! Another small but significant change is Addie's newly found sensitivity to loud
sounds and moods. She used to sleep through the activity
in the house, and I encouraged everyone to keep the noise
level normal and not to tiptoe around her. But recently,

noises interrupt her sleep. At night she will go back down with no interference on our part, but during naps, once awakened, she stays awake. Addie functions best with a short morning nap and a long afternoon nap, but she has been having problems lately with her afternoon nap. One problem I discovered was that her room was too bright. I started to notice she would sleep soundly on cloudy days, but on sunny days, when her room is very bright, she would awaken with a screech. Her room faces south and with white walls, the reflection is startling, even when the blinds are closed. Once I dropped something in her room, and she howled inconsolably. I guess nap times can't always be perfect.

The most surprising response was when I leaned over her cribside one day, and with a mock frown stated in a serious tone, "You should be sleeping, Miss Kishbaugh." She eyed me suspiciously and broke into sobs. Crying also closely follows laughing sometimes; the emotional swings of a baby can be confusing. At times like these, I just call her my little Eve and give her an extra hug and a kiss.

On a less cheerful note, Addie's last pneumogram showed that she needs to continue on the monitor for at least three more months until she receives two good consecutive tests. Oddly enough, her heart rate was fine, but they felt that she had had too many episodes of inconsistent breathing periods to consider removing her from the monitor. All babies have these breathing periods, but Addie is a bit above the 5 percent limit that is set for children of her age. We were disappointed, but philosophical. We will do what we have to do, of course. At this point, using the monitor is so routine that we barely notice it. Addie is safe and happy and growing nicely, and *that* is what matters most.

Dad's Thoughts

Addie and I have been talking a lot lately, which becomes noteworthy when you realize that she has no vocabulary whatsoever. Babies, of course, communicate from birth.

But Adelyn has reached the age when she is experimenting with her voice and beginning to develop less instinctive, more cognitive communication. In addition to telling us when she is hungry or tired or angry, she tells us when she is bored or contented or even when she is busy with one of her toys.

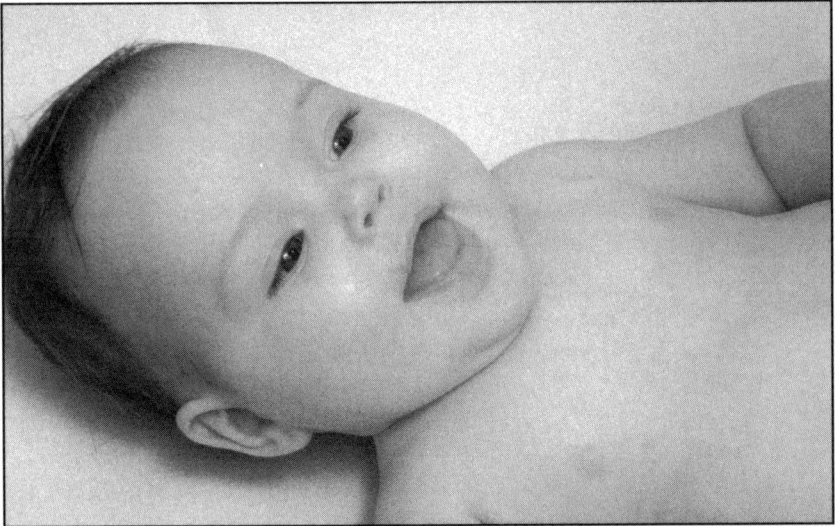

Addie enjoys babbling, especially when it is naked playtime.

Addie lies in her crib or her playpen and "talks." She coos, gurgles, and hoots. That last, "hoots," is the name I've ascribed to those times when her voice pops out of her with such force that even she is surprised. By practicing, she has developed variations in inflection. I notice this because I have been able to spend more time with her lately. Since Ann has resumed her freelance writing career and is now working on a steady basis, I've been helping pick up the slack, feeding, changing, and playing with Addie more. Addie responds to my voice with hers, and the exchange has begun to resemble a conversation. I surprise her by varying the timing and inflection of my words. This usually elicits giggles and continued responses. Addie is particularly talkative in those places she is most secure like her crib, play-pen, and changing table—especially the changing table. Annie and I often change her together and, with both of us there, it becomes a real social situation, perhaps a precursor to the dinnertime family hour.

This brings me to what is probably the most dramatic change in Addie's routine—solid food. Ann had noticed Addie watching us eat. It is one of the classic clues that indicates a child is ready for this step. When Annie decided to introduce solid food, she made sure I was there with the camera. We were expecting, with a sort of sadistic anticipation, the "yech" response. We set up the infant seat, I got

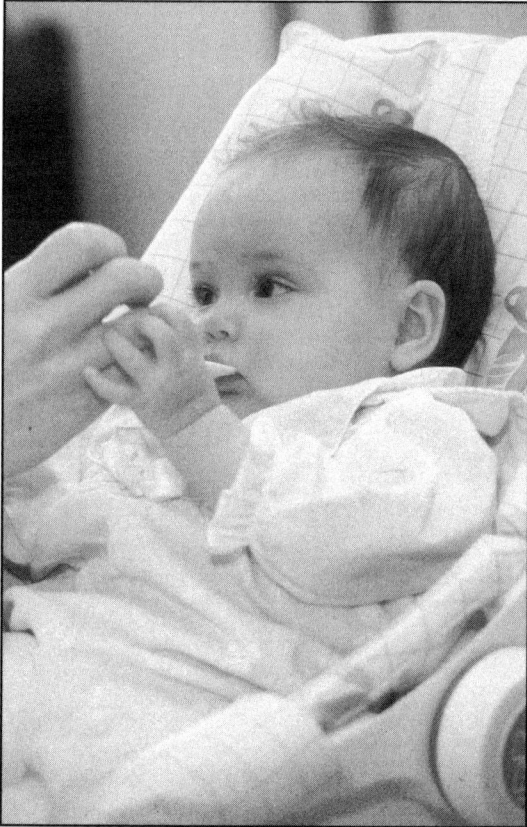

Adelyn loved her first taste of "real" food.

my photography equipment together, placed Addie in the seat, smashed the banana, and donned foul-weather gear. She loved it. With the first spoonful, she grabbed Ann's hand and pulled it toward her mouth. Okay, we thought, so she likes bananas. They are sweet and the consistency is fun to play with. Just wait until we try vegetables, Addie.

Well, that day came, and as before, Ann insisted I have the camera ready. Addie was in her seat and the veggies were waiting. As Ann pushed the first spoonful toward her, I focused the lens. (You should now be hearing the shark music from *Jaws*.) Again, no luck. She loved them. In fact, she loves everything we try. She slurps it up as fast as we can spoon it to her, although the barley and prunes I gave her for breakfast this morning slowed her down a bit. All in all though, this thirteen-pounder is becoming a real chow hound.

I remember writing a few months ago that I looked forward to the day when Ann and I were more equal partners in caring for Addie. With Annie working more and Addie taking solid food, that day has come. The fact that we both work from home allows us this luxury of sharing in her care. It is a luxury that seems not only natural but more efficient as well. By far the greatest benefit is the additional time I get to spend with my little girl.

Sixth Month—Pediatric Commentary by Dr. Marie Keith

Having carefully mastered breast or bottle-feeding, most parents of a six-month-old are eager to embark on a new feeding adventure—the introduction of solid foods. The trend in infant feeding has changed over the years. Current thinking promotes the introduction of solid food feedings sometime between three and six months.

There are many factors that help determine when an infant is ready for this new experience. The baby should be able to hold her head up steadily in a sitting position. Like Addie Ruth, many babies also show obvious interest in the process of eating as they carefully watch their parents take each bite of food.

There also are physiological signs to watch for such as frequent feeding during the day or reappearance of night wakings for feeding when the baby previously slept through the night. In their own time, babies begin to have increased caloric needs for growth based on their levels of activity and mobility and their individual metabolic rates. Breastfed babies may markedly increase their nursing activity. Babies who are formula-fed may consume much larger amounts of formula, up to thirty-five to forty ounces a day. Some infants who are exclusively breastfed begin to show a drop-off in growth rate as their needs for calories surpass the mother's rate of milk production.

The reasons to delay introducing solid foods must be weighed against the signs of your baby's readiness and physiological needs. A strong family history of allergy or early signs of allergy in the baby (such as eczema) would warrant waiting until about six months of age for solid foods. The immature digestive tract may allow protein allergens to pass into the baby's system setting up sensitivities that could lead to short-or long-term allergy problems. If the baby experienced digestive difficulty such as colic in the early months, it also may be better to postpone beginning solid food

feedings. Some infants who show excessive weight gain in the early months also may grow more evenly with delayed introduction of solids and addition of more water to their diets.

It's important to begin adding solid foods slowly. In the first weeks of feeding, the baby needs to learn how to get the food off the spoon and into the back of her mouth and then how to swallow it. This sounds like a simple procedure, but until now, the baby has dealt only with sucking and swallowing a liquid and needs some measure of practice to learn. Also, the baby's digestive system is accustomed only to processing a liquid diet and too much solid food at once could certainly lead to indigestion. In the first month of feeding, one meal a day is recommended. The timing is not crucial, but consistency in time is important. Many parents prefer to feed their babies one meal of solid food in the evening, hoping to achieve better nighttime sleep patterns. The quantity of food in the first weeks of feeding should be small—one tablespoon to begin, then an increasing amount as the baby shows the ability or eagerness to take more.

Although some pediatricians suggest starting with a fruit, generally the first food is a cereal grain—rice, oatmeal, or barley baby cereal. Cereals for babies are iron fortified to help provide for the infant's increasing need for this mineral. Initially the cereal should be mixed to a fairly thin consistency with a few ounces of fluid, either breast milk, formula, water, or juice. Feed the cereal mixture with a small spoon. A feeding dish that warms the cereal slightly is a useful feeding aid.

The baby may at first show some difficulty handling solid food in her mouth. It helps to scoop the food off the spoon onto the roof of the baby's mouth, from where she can lick it with her tongue. Much of the food may be thrust forward with the tongue onto the lips or forcefully spit out! At first you and the baby may be wearing more food than you'd like. Gently regather the food about the lips and reintroduce it. After the first week or two of feedings, the baby gradually learns how to handle the solid food and readily opens up for the next spoonful. At this point, you can increase the quantity of food to the amount the baby seems to want. Babies usually clearly signal when they want more or when they've had enough.

Adding variety is the next step. As a general guideline, introducing one new food each week is a good policy. This allows the parent to assess any adverse effects the baby may experience with a particular food. The signs of digestive difficulties are vomiting, diarrhea, excessive gassiness, or severe constipation. Skin rashes such as blotchy hives or eczema also indicate that a food is not right for your baby. When new foods are intro-

duced singly and gradually, you can isolate the food that is causing the adverse reaction and eliminate it.

After cereal, a pureed fruit or vegetable is the next choice. To aid in the digestive process, most fruits or vegetables should be cooked and pureed to a thin consistency. Prepared baby food in jars or home cooked fruits or vegetables pureed in a blender make exciting new meals. Fruits that usually are readily digested are mashed ripe banana, applesauce, pears, peaches, or plums. Yellow vegetables such as carrots, squash, or sweet potatoes also are good choices. Solid foods in the diet will make some changes in the color and consistency of the stools. Iron fortification of cereal may produce a dark green or black color. Partially digested food particles may come through in the color of the food eaten.

During the early months of your baby's experience with solid foods, breast or formula feeding continues without dramatic change. When second and third meals are introduced a few months later, the breast or bottle feedings may decrease as the baby receives increasing nutrition from solid foods.

Introducing solid food is a fun but messy experience for everyone involved. It allows the baby to experiment with new tastes and textures and with an exciting new activity—playing with food. It is a true adventure!

Fourth through Sixth Months—Child Development Commentary by Dr. Anita Hurtig

Something wonderful and exciting is happening to Addie in her fourth month of life. Ann describes it as Addie's efforts to "reach out more to the world"; Nevin has her "becoming more social." Starting at three to four months and extending to six months we find the infant taking a dramatic leap into the social world. Ann perceives this in a range of behaviors, including staring, searching for reactions, reaching, grasping, and smiling. Here we see the subtle, constant, and essential interplay between motor action and mental interaction. As Addie gains sensori-motor skills, she builds the structures, or what Piaget calls schema, for control and activation of herself and the important people in her world. Smiling is the most powerful activator a baby has, an essential social tool in the ongoing duet between parent and infant. The smile serves to both communicate the baby's inner state and to cue the parent toward empathic responses.

But it is not only in these non-vocal behaviors that Addie reveals her social awareness and control. The beginning of vocalization—babbling—is the blossoming of socialization. Ann correctly describes this as a "dialogue" between mother and infant, a dialogue which is basic to the communication they both work so hard to achieve—mother by finding the right tone, the right pace, the right melody—infant by responding with her own tones, smiles and body movement.

In these soulful interactions, Ann and Addie are working to help Addie structure her social world, construct a world of people. Through this construction Addie increasingly becomes aware of the joys and the dangers inherent in social interaction. The joys are abundant, as exemplified in Ann's glowing description of Addie's ingratiating laugh. Addie's laugh successfully draws her mother's attention, as if to say, "hi, I'm here—look at me." But the hazards of social interaction are real, as evidenced by Addie's reaction to the roughness of her mother's voice which indicated some danger that the warm and predictable bond can be shattered. The hazards are also experienced in the presence of a new and unfamiliar face whose details and sound and movement don't conform to the comforting familiar presences. Only because the infant is actively constructing a social world of safe and trusted presences can some be experienced as unsafe. Thus, the classic six month stranger anxiety, the hallmark of both connectedness and differentiation.

85

Nevin, too, senses some highly significant change is occurring. He characterizes Addie as "beginning to realize who we were" and thus leaving infancy and entering babyhood. He speaks of Ann and Addie's "interdependence." Ann sees this as a time of "first letting go," of growing differentiation which is both exciting and frightening, a push-pull which Ann will experience throughout Addie's development and which will demand sensitive negotiation through the shoals of holding on and pushing away, for both child and parent(s). Addie's actions and reactions, her smiling and reaching out, her manipulation of objects (human and otherwise) to get them to respond to her, and her ability to hold and retrieve attention by staring, looking away, looking back, are components of what developmentalists call a sense of self. Self-hood for Addie means that she and her mother and father are separate, but impact on one another in powerful and effective ways. Child developmentalists have long been concerned with the question of when an infant begins to differentiate, that is, have a sense that their *self* is a separate entity from their entire universe of experience, to "decenter" in Piaget's terms. Until very recently the common assumption has been that the first nine months or so of an infant's life are a state of "normal symbioses," a kind of fusion in which figure (self) and ground (everything else) is a single, undifferentiated mass of feeling. Current infant research, based on careful physiological and observational data, indicates that differentiation is accomplished much earlier, even as early as three to four months and into the sixth month. Ann and Nevin's vigilance and sensitivity support these observations.

In a recent book on how the baby's interpersonal world develops, Daniel Stern describes the many facets of this world. He defines four characteristics of this period which are essential to the development of a sense of a "core" self and relatedness. These are 1) self-agency, the baby's sense of volition and control; 2) self-coherence, the baby's sense of physical wholeness; 3) self-affectivity, the baby's inner qualities and feeling; and 4) self-history, the baby's inner sense of continuity. Addie demonstrates these in her smiles, her variable responsivity, her motivation to master and control. These are the building blocks for what we will see developing in the next few months as Addie not only senses her own and others' unique wholeness, but becomes aware that she can share this "core" with others, and they with her. Without these qualities Addie would remain severely impaired, unresponsive and attentive only to her own needs and impulses, limited to an "autistic" world of self-involvement.

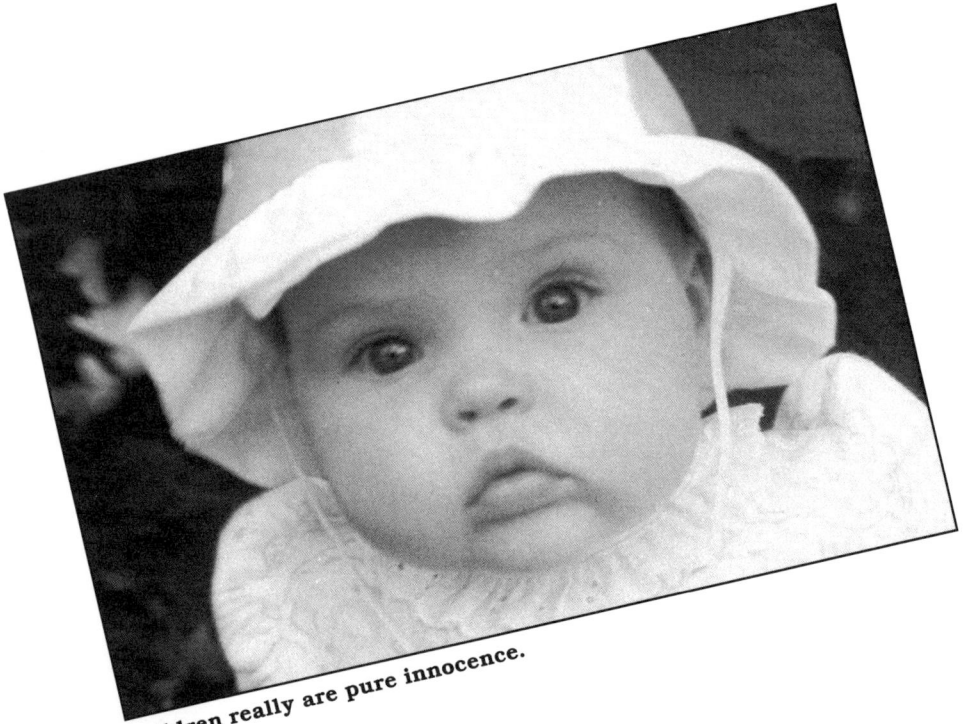

Children really are pure innocence.

Seventh Month

Mom's Thoughts

At the doctor's office for her six-month check-up, Addie was much happier than she had been at her last visit. She accepted the DPT shot like an old pro, and her tears dried quickly. We reached a milestone this month: Addie's height and weight are now on the charts! She is in the tenth percentile for weight and the thirtieth percentile for height. The main topic of conversation between the doctor and me this time was food. On our last visit when Addie was four months old, we briefly discussed introducing solids in very small amounts, but now that we were ready to do more than just taste, I was looking for more guidance in increasing her intake. So I left the doctor's office with lots of notes about feeding Addie, including new foods she now could try as well as the amounts.

I've read that between the ages of six and eight months, all babies are busy doing *something*. Adelyn has been very physical this month. She's currently busy strengthening the muscles that she will use to sit alone. When breastfeeding, Adelyn will stop and pull herself up to a sitting position (at least as much as she can manage without assistance). Some days when she is feeling quite powerful, she can sit up in one swift movement; but most days she needs help when she gets about halfway there. Breastfeeding now takes an inordinate amount of time (except for her first feeding that is ravenously taken at 6:00 A.M.). Feed. Sit up. Feed. Sit up. Adelyn is like a yo-yo.

When Addie first started trying to do this, I was at my wit's end because I couldn't figure out what it was she wanted. She would stop nursing, throw her head back, then try hard to pull her head back up to the breast. She'd complain and squirm. I was baffled. I thought perhaps she liked looking at the world upside down, but didn't understand what all this commotion was about? Was it gas? Teething? Wasn't there enough milk? Eventually, the clues added up and mother figured it out. This happens a lot these days.

Adelyn also likes tearing apart her playpen and crib. She readily picks up and examines various toys, discarding them when they bore her. Frequently, I look down into her crib and have trouble finding her in the chaos of toys, stuffed animals, blanket, arms, and legs. She can swivel around almost 180 degrees on her back or on her stomach (when she will accept this position). When Addie is on her stomach, she can easily play with toys in front of her and is learning how to pull them within her grasp. She can roll over from either position, but she hasn't been that interested in pursuing this activity. Instead she prefers reaching way back from either side to grope for the toy that she

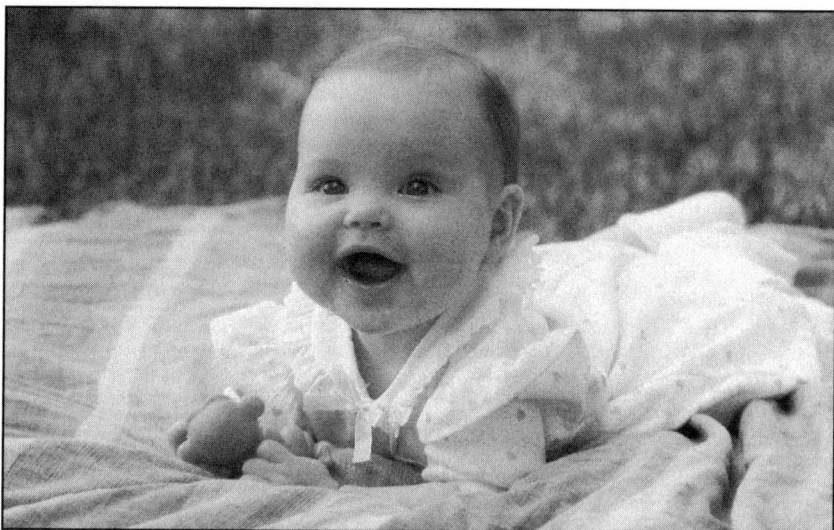

That toy in her hand is one of the ugliest toys I've ever seen, but Addie loves it—especially its "squeak."

wants. Her legs shuffle back and forth, but she still shows no signs of trying to get up onto her knees and crawl forward. Continue those powerful leg thrusts, Addie!

Adelyn is not yet an accomplished sitter, but will be any day now. She can balance for a short time, but still topples easily. Each day, however, we are seeing improvement in her balancing act. She is now using the high chair (my sister gave me the key to this: put a foam rubber pad underneath her to prevent slipping and then strap her in) and likes playing with things on her tray. But when she's eating in the high chair, she throws her arms back as though someone said, "Stick'em up, Adelyn." She also does this when she is sitting on my hip. The only conclusion I can draw is that she is balancing herself with the help of her arms.

When Addie is eating, if I'm too slow in getting the food to her, she will grab the spoon herself and poke at her face with it. Sometimes she even manages to find her mark. Everything placed on her tray eventually finds its way to her mouth or more likely, to the floor. She loves eating—and, I've discovered, watching Mom work.

The arrival of hot weather and her increased physical activity have introduced a few other problems. Since Adelyn has been wearing only T-shirts to bed, she has discovered the wires that attach her to the heart monitor, which are great fun to play with. She twists and turns with them in her hands and eventually pulls them loose. We are now awakened by the lead alarm at 5:00 A.M. when Addie has decided to play before she is fed. (A lead alarm is a continuous alarm that indicates a system problem as opposed to the staccato beeps that indicate a breathing problem.) When I enter her room in response to the alarm, I find Addie looking at her wires with deep concentration. Then, when she sees me, she gives me a big grin. Coincidentally, I have recently heard stories of children who pull the wires out deliberately for attention. Pull the wire, hear the alarm, then watch for mom or dad.

A wonderful recent development is Addie's growing interest in her sense of touch. I first noticed this early in the month when she began stroking my breast when she was feeding. She would glide her hand back and forth ever so gently. It was a welcome change from the grab and twist phase of last month.

At times, she'll pull our faces down to hers and gently suck (kiss?) on our noses or chins while stroking our faces. Addie also enthusiastically throws her arms around us almost like a big hug and strokes the back of our necks lightly, a gesture that just melts our hearts.

I frequently use a tissue to clean her face after she spits up, and one time she picked up a tissue that was lying around and instead of shoving it into her mouth, as she does with everything else, she wiped her face with it. Crumpling newspapers and magazines is a favorite pastime. If we are out and about and I need to amuse her for a few minutes, I can always find a magazine for her.

Addie also enjoys our bedtime ritual of reading to her. She actually prefers some books to others. If she doesn't like a book, she'll squirm and complain, but as soon as I pick up a book she likes, she settles down. She smiles as soon as she sees Big Bird and also smiles in anticipation of what will be said. When we reach the page on which I say "Peeka-boo," she turns her face around and looks up at me expectantly. A few months ago she seemed interested only in the pages and in helping me turn them, but now, the repetition of the content is what fascinates her. I gave her a board book to take to bed with her the other day, and she had a great time looking at the pages and turning them until sleep overcame her and her thumb beckoned her to put the book down.

Addie's latest interest is putting her fingers into our mouths when we are talking to her. She does this fre-

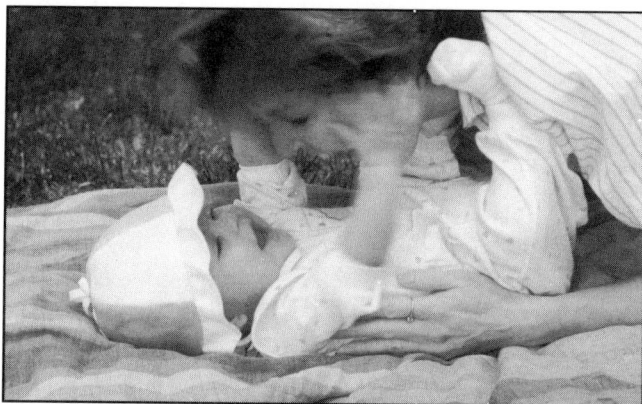

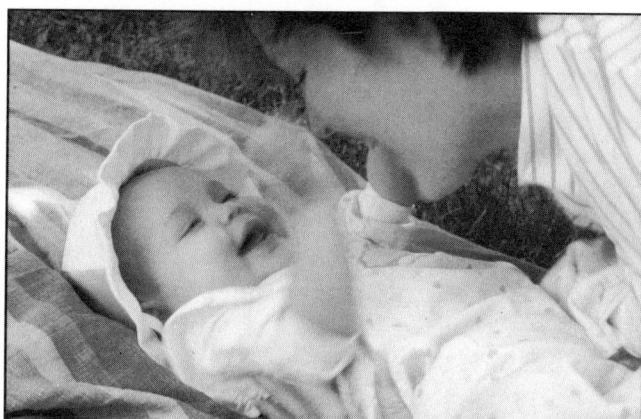

Playing with Annie. There are some moments that are magic—this was one of them.

quently and gets a big charge out of it. Singing into her fingers intrigues her. Sometimes she will respond to us softly, and lately she has started talking while nursing. Her sounds now seem to be more complex in that they're not always just one sound repeated over and over, but a combination of sounds with various inflections. You almost get the sense that there is a flow of conversation to them. She listens with rapt attention when Nevin and I are having a conversation near her.

Sometimes, Addie finds a totally new sound to practice. One night after we put her to bed, Nevin and I had a great time listening to Addie learn to blow out with her lips pursued. She spent a half hour learning this new technique. When the house finally grew quiet again, Nevin turned to me and said, "You know what this means don't you? Food will never stay in her mouth again."

Dad's Thoughts

As Addie reaches the end of her sixth month, she is slowly making progress in motor development. While she has excellent control of her hands —she switches toys from hand to hand, grasps desired objects easily (including my nose and mustache) and, with a little effort, reaches virtually anything in her playpen—in two areas, she has not accomplished as much as we expected her to accomplish. She can roll over but does so only to avoid being on her stomach. Also, while her back is strong—strong enough to support her—she really does not like to sit upright. I know that all children develop these skills at their own pace, and I understand logically that there is absolutely no reason to be concerned. But still, it is a subject we've talked about, and we, like most new parents, I'm sure, wonder if we are doing enough for her.

In fact, we've been actively trying to spur her advancement in this area. Through repeated attempts, she has learned to play on her stomach for short periods. Not only has this given her a new perspective on the world, it has helped to improve her coordination. Addie, while on her stomach, supports her weight on her elbows and reaches for and plays with the toys placed in front of her. Now, when she rolls onto her back, it is with deliberate motion rather than a combination of anger and accident.

As a result of her improved hand/eye coordination, Adelyn has made an important discovery: hands are not just for grasping. For one thing, they can *feel*—my unshaven face in the morning or the dogs' soft fur and cold, wet noses. I'm not sure if her newly found fascination with dogs led to the discovery of their texture, or if she developed interest in them after finding out that they felt nice. But she definitely likes them. She looks for them when she hears their nails clicking on the wood floors. When one of them comes into view, she smiles and reaches out. They oblige and come closer. Addie strokes their fur and smiles. I can see them becoming fast friends in a few years. She'll benefit by never being without a playmate, and they, well, any food she eats will be at their eye level—and that has to be appealing.

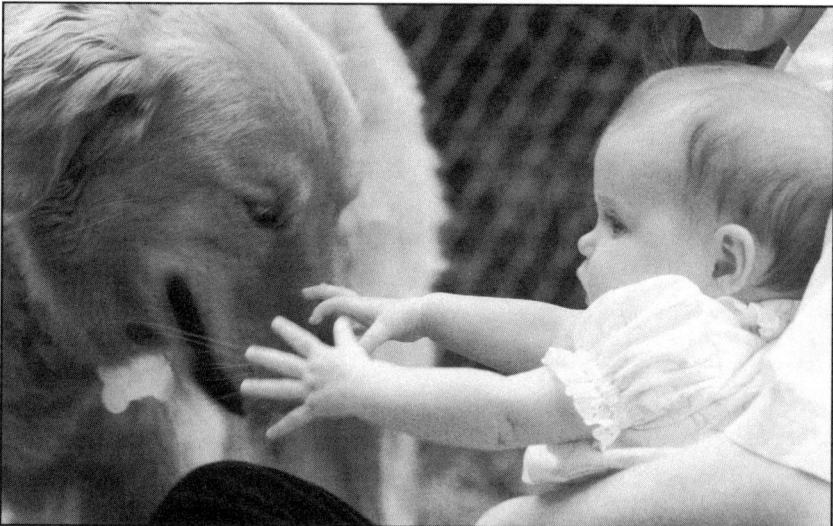

Adelyn and Beau have become great friends, despite the fact that he's still a little jealous of her.

Hands also show affection, and Addie has been show-ing her affection for us. She'll stroke the back of Ann's neck or her cheek gently and deliberately. Sometimes she will take Ann's face in her hands and "kiss" her. It's not a tradi-tional kiss, with pursed lips, but more of a "chew." She opens her mouth wide and sort of gums Ann's cheek or chin (which gives new meaning to the phrase "suck face"). She does this in direct response to our kisses, and it is the most gratifying and touching of all her gestures.

On those occasions when I'm home in the afternoon, I like to take Addie for a walk in her stroller. She likes to be outside; she watches the flicker of sunlight through the

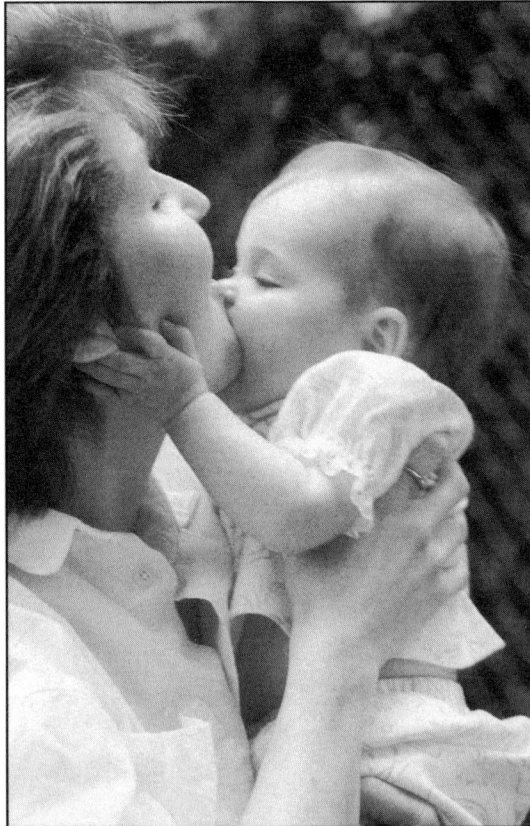

A "kiss" for Annie.

trees, and she loves to watch cars go by. As the sound of one approaches, she turns to look for it. When she finds it, she seems to lock in on it, following it with her eyes as it rolls past and up the street. When one car stopped in front of a house ahead of us and a man got out, she seemed a little surprised. I don't think she has made the connection between the car we get into and the ones she sees on the street.

It's not far from our house to the park, where there are swings, slides, see-saws, and kids—lots of kids. Addie and I sit on one of the benches and just watch awhile. She loves to watch the kids play (so do I). There is constant movement. The younger ones bounce from the slide to the swings to the jungle gym and back again. Boys wrestle on the ground and chase each other, playing "keep away" with somebody's shoe. Older girls, nearing their teens, gather in groups and whisper and giggle. Addie's eyes seem to take in every movement. A squeal or laughter catches her attention, and she shifts her eyes to meet it. She holds my hand.

I wonder if she knows it will be her turn soon.

Seventh Month—Pediatric Commentary by Dr. Marie Keith

Unabashed joy and wonderment are the key words that describe the disposition of a baby entering the seventh month. Each day holds the promise of new adventure and new accomplishments. The baby's behavior is typified by a restless energy that is an outgrowth of all the excitement she feels as she discovers new and wonderful things about the world around her. Addie's response to the family pets, her parents' conversations, the world inside her crib and outside the house are all evidence of this excitement.

Most infants at this age like to greet the day at or near dawn —often to the dismay of their tired parents. Like other creatures up at this hour, they also like to chirp and may be heard babbling contentedly in their cribs for the first half hour or so, until they begin to demand some attention.

By this stage in development, babies' vocalizations have become quite varied. They can express themselves at many different pitches and intensities. The open-mouthed vowel sounds are emitted as yells and squeals. They begin experimenting with different positions of the tongue and lips, and produce various consonant sounds. Many babies find that covering and uncovering their mouth with the hand makes an interesting sound effect and practice this maneuver at length. Babies love to have people converse with them and make the same sounds they make. Babbling is an important preliminary to language development and baby talk is fun for adults. too.

The baby's hands and mouth are the primary means of exploration, so much so that even a casual observer of a seven-month-old will notice she brings everything to her mouth. Reaching for objects with the whole hand and a palm grasp has been perfected. Now she begins to explore with the fingers. Her fingertips touch tiny objects —buttons, threads, crumbs— and attempt to pick them up as she practices the pincer grasp, which uses the index finger and the thumb.

A word of caution is needed here. As babies begin to be able to pick up small items, which they then bring to their mouths, there is the potential for choking accidents. Another significant danger for babies at this age, brought about by the developing use of the hands, is scald burns caused by reaching for a hot cup of coffee, tea or soup. So parents must become very vigilant.

In addition to oral exploration, another reason babies bring objects to their mouths is to massage their gums. Most babies teethe at this age. Exactly what a baby feels is hard to know, but clearly there is a change in sensation in the gums that leads a baby to want to chew on anything in sight. Teething babies salivate or drool excessively and like to protrude their tongues over the lower gum and suck in their lower lips over the gum. Oftentimes, teething babies have unexpected crying spells that seem to stem from pain in the gums. Teething pain can be relieved by a teething toy, a cool wash cloth, a topical anesthetic made for teething, or the judicious use of an oral analgesic such as acetaminophen.

Teething also may interrupt a previously well-established night sleeping pattern. As the baby enters the lighter phase of the sleep cycle, throbbing pain in the gums may begin to produce night wakings. Another source of restless sleep at this stage probably derives from more lively dream content. The baby may be reliving some of the day's activities in her dream sleep and be much more restless during these dream cycles. It is helpful at this point to settle the baby back to sleep with as little intervention as possible so that her nighttime sleep patterns may be maintained. Usually some gentle soothing is all that is needed.

Two of the accomplishments that babies probably dream about are progress toward sitting and crawling. Most infants at this age will attempt to come forward to you as you reach to pick them up. This development accompanies strengthening of their back and abdominal muscles, and they usually sit quite comfortably propped against you or in the corner of a soft chair or couch. When they begin to be able to sit somewhat on their own, it's usually in the awkward tripod position in which they lean far forward, supporting themselves with both hands and their buttocks. As their balance beings to improve and the muscles of their backs strengthen, they develop a more upright posture and are able to right themselves when they list from side to side. Once they can balance, the hands are free to engage in other activities while sitting.

Early attempts at crawling are like a comedy of errors. Motivated by something in her sight, the baby tries to move forward. Usually her arms are more coordinated than her legs at this point and in pushing with the arms, she usually propels herself backwards. When her knees finally come up under her abdomen, she might practice a rocking motion that often leads to many falls forward onto the face! But with diligent tenacity, the baby tries again and again and finally begins to inch forward using a coordinated movement of hands and legs and slowly a true crawl evolves.

The seven-month-old is on the brink of many achievements. You can see in each baby this age a sense of striving to master a task and frustration at failure. There is a delightful display of self-esteem and happiness in accomplishment, which makes this an especially sweet time to watch your baby grow.

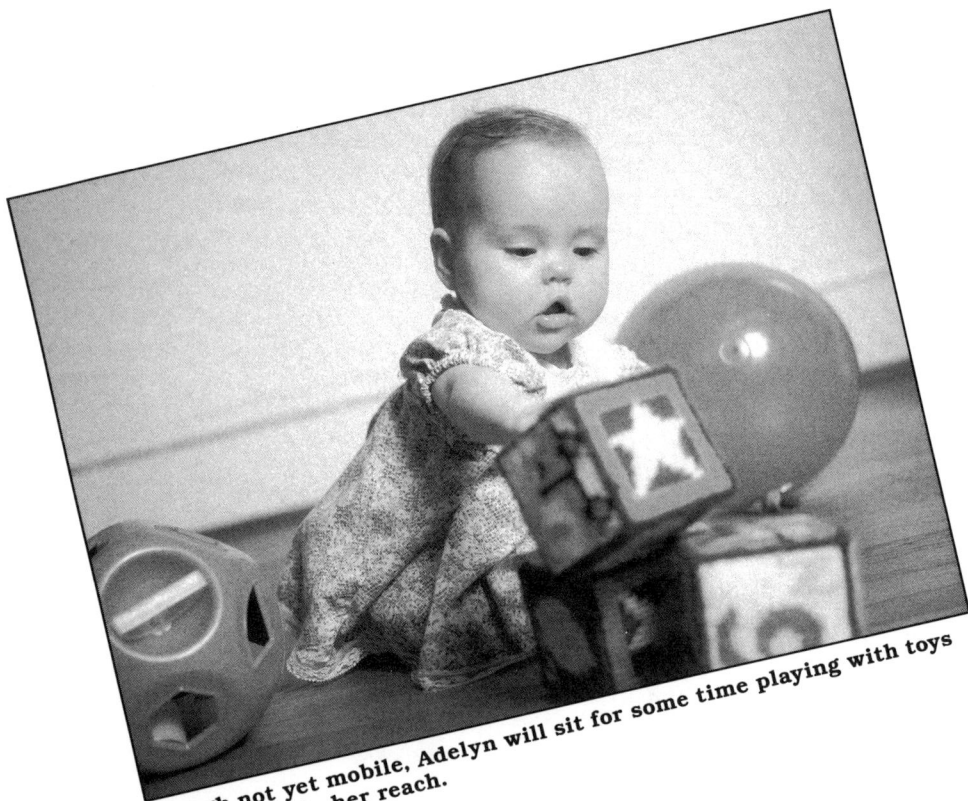

Though not yet mobile, Adelyn will sit for some time playing with toys that are within her reach.

Eighth Month

Mom's Thoughts

All of Adelyn's exercising has paid off. She can now sit unsupported and play with toys within her reach. I was surprised to discover that she had this ability one night when she was taking a bath. Up until that time, she would sit rather precariously in the tub, swaying from side to side after a minute or two. On this particular night, however, I set her in the tub and noticed she seemed steadier than she had previously. My hands wavered around her waiting for the inevitable side sway, but it never came. She reached out in front of her, grabbed a toy floating by in the shallow water, and raised it to her mouth. I was so excited for her. I could tell she was impressed, too, because she was braver than usual and after a time, tried to lunge toward a floating toy. It wasn't exactly the time to try lunging, but with some help she ended up on her belly and tried to crawl, only she did it backwards and ended up at the other end of the tub! It's a start.

As with the backward crawling, Adelyn is experimenting with different methods of locomotion. When she is on her stomach, she digs her toes into the carpet and tries to push herself forward. Her rear end raises appropriately, but she hasn't yet figured out the motions that accompany it, so a lot of frustrated yelling ensues.

Adelyn loves her walker. Let me rephrase that: Adelyn now loves her walker. When I first put her into it, she went backward which really scared her. She cried in terror, so we put the walker away for another day. It took a few tries but once she became accustomed to it, she found the new vantage point a nice change from the floor. Addie started crowing excitedly whenever we put her in it. She moved her feet underneath her, first in sheer excitement and then with slow purpose. This new ambulatory ability has opened her world considerably.

We often go out to the sidewalk that leads to our house, and Addie yells in delight from her walker at whomever passes (she loves to try out different pitches this month), bangs her toys on her tray, fingers all of the plants that are at her height in the front garden (but I have to be very careful that there is no tasting as plants can be very poisonous), and performs her favorite activity—watching the progress of every vehicle that goes up or down our street. I label them for her. "Here comes the truck, Addie." "See the motorcycle." She watches each one with furrowed eyebrows.

I have recently been hearing and reading a lot about the dangers of children and walkers. Nevin and I are very careful about our use of this device, and as Addie becomes more proficient, we will have to be extra vigilant, and, per-

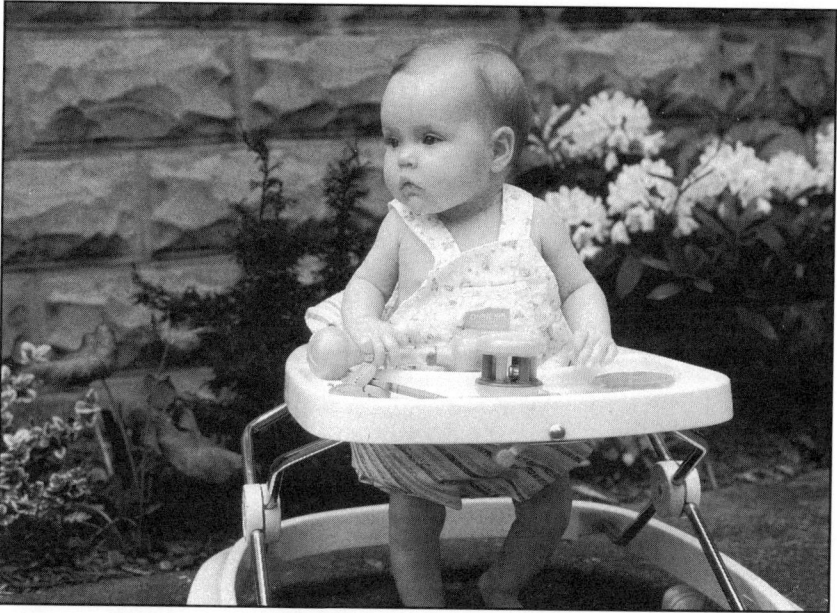

Adelyn enjoying her favorite activity—watching the progress of every vehicle that goes up or down our street.

haps, reevaluate our use of it. But, for now, the walker provides Addie with a great sense of accomplishment.

Another favorite activity is eating Cheerios. I have been fascinated with the development of her coordination. At first, she would grab fistfuls and then suck her thumb to get the flavor. (The Cheerios would turn to mush in her palm.) Then she realized they were sticking to her fingertips or her hand, and she would raise her hand slowly to her mouth, all the while keeping her mouth open expectantly. (I would be sitting and watching her with baited breath.) Once she realized that she could apply the pincer grasp (thumb and index finger), she began picking them up, and very slowly and carefully bringing them to her mouth. (You could tell it was the most delicate of operations.)

Sometimes she would lean her mouth down so that it almost touched the tray. Using this technique, she doesn't have to raise her hand so far and perhaps be unsuccessful in getting the Cheerio to its target. After she put the Cheerio in her mouth, however, she didn't realize that she had to let it go! I would breathe a sign of relief that she had accomplished her task, and out would pop her fingers with the soggy Cheerio in them. She would look puzzled, then she would suck her thumb (more for comfort, I believe) which solved the problem. The Cheerio would dissolve in her mouth.

Adelyn also has been learning to use her hands in more complex ways. When I suggest "shake, shake, shake," she will sometimes shake the object she is holding in her hand —and grin. She is also trying to clap her hands and do "pat-

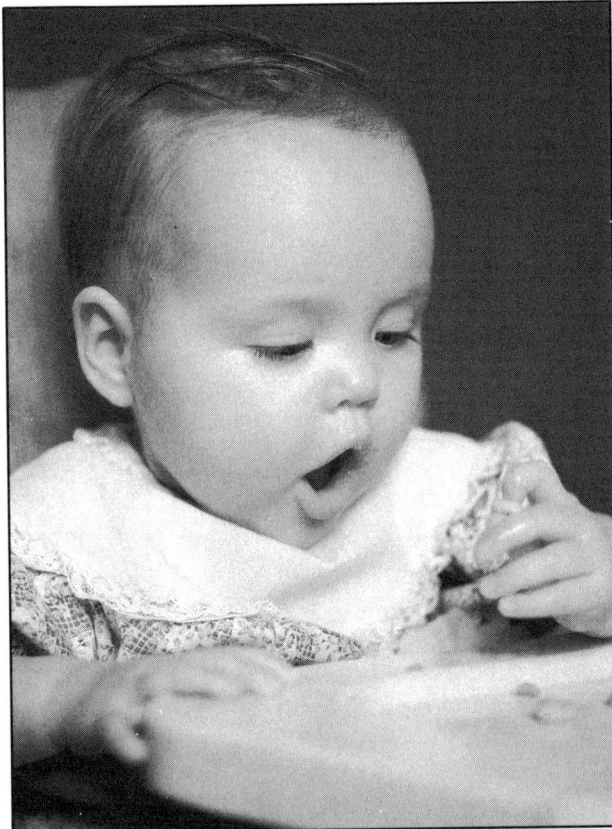

The "pincer grasp" is a learned art; the Cheerios®, of course, are great motivation.

tycake," sometimes at my suggestion but more often independently. Her hands don't often meet, but she is trying. Addie likes the song, "When You're Happy and You Know It Clap Your Hands," although she'd rather watch me than do it herself. She's also using her hands more to indicate what she wants, such as her cup or bottle of juice.

Two very important milestones happened on the same day. First, at seven and one-half months of age, Addie finally came off of the heart monitor. She passed her pneumogram with flying colors. We eagerly disconnected the machine after we received the telephone call and looked forward (although a tiny bit apprehensively) to our first solo night. We

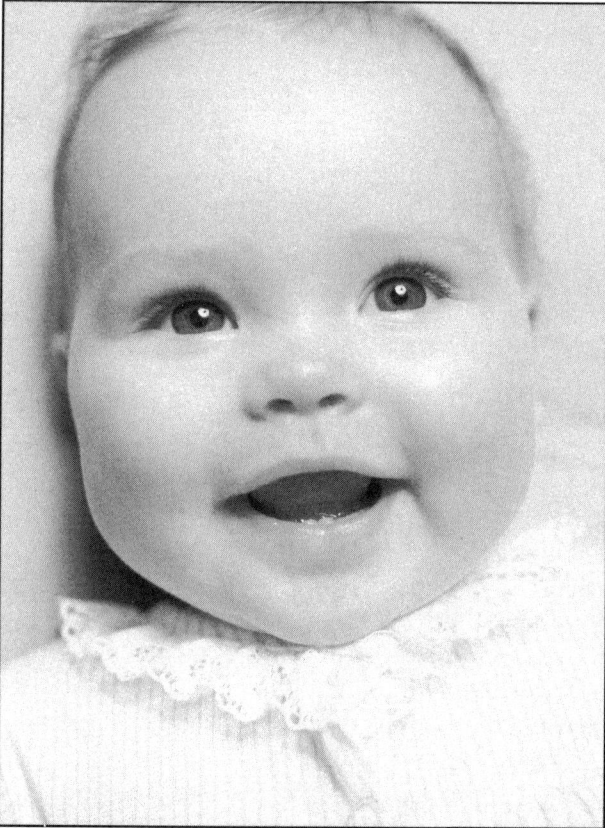

Showing off her brand new teeth.

didn't have to worry about checking on her, however. She checked in with us every hour: it was teething night.

To her credit, Addie handled it very well. (I understand that if adults had the same pain, it would feel about ten times worse.) She fussed every hour but didn't really cry out for attention until 2:00 A.M. At that point, she really let loose, and when Dad went in to her room to comfort her, lo and behold he found her first tooth, the second major event in less than twenty-four hours. A little teething gel, some Infant's Tylenol, some hugs and kisses, and a lullaby took care of the worst of it, and she was back to bed within the hour. Two days later, the second tooth appeared much more quietly than the first. She now has a matched set on the bottom front row. When she went to gum my nose and bit it instead, she was very surprised when I cried out. And, of course, she tried out her new teeth while nursing. Suffice it to say, she now knows the meaning of "No!"

Another important event is Adelyn's first weaning since she gave up the late night feeding four months ago. Adelyn has been on four feedings a day for a while, but I noticed recently that she would play around at the mid-morning nursing as if she wasn't that interested but be ravenous by 2:00 P.M. So I tried cutting out the second feeding and moved her lunch up to 11:30 A.M. Addie now eats heartily at each meal. With the addition of a variety of solid foods to her diet, a three-meal-a-day schedule suits her well. I have found that a teething biscuit (Adelyn loves them but are they messy!) and some juice after her afternoon nap help her to wait until 5:00 P.M. for her dinner. (Five hours is a long time to go without something to tide you over.) Since the weaning was gradual (she lessened her intake over a couple of days), I had little discomfort. I was surprised to find that I experienced little sense of loss (perhaps the biting had something to do with that!). Instead, I feel proud that my little girl is growing up, and I'm also enjoying the extra freedom it provides me.

Addie has been laughing a lot this month. She chuckles at Dad as he plays with his Nerf basketball in the living room. She laughs at Grandfather Kishbaugh when he

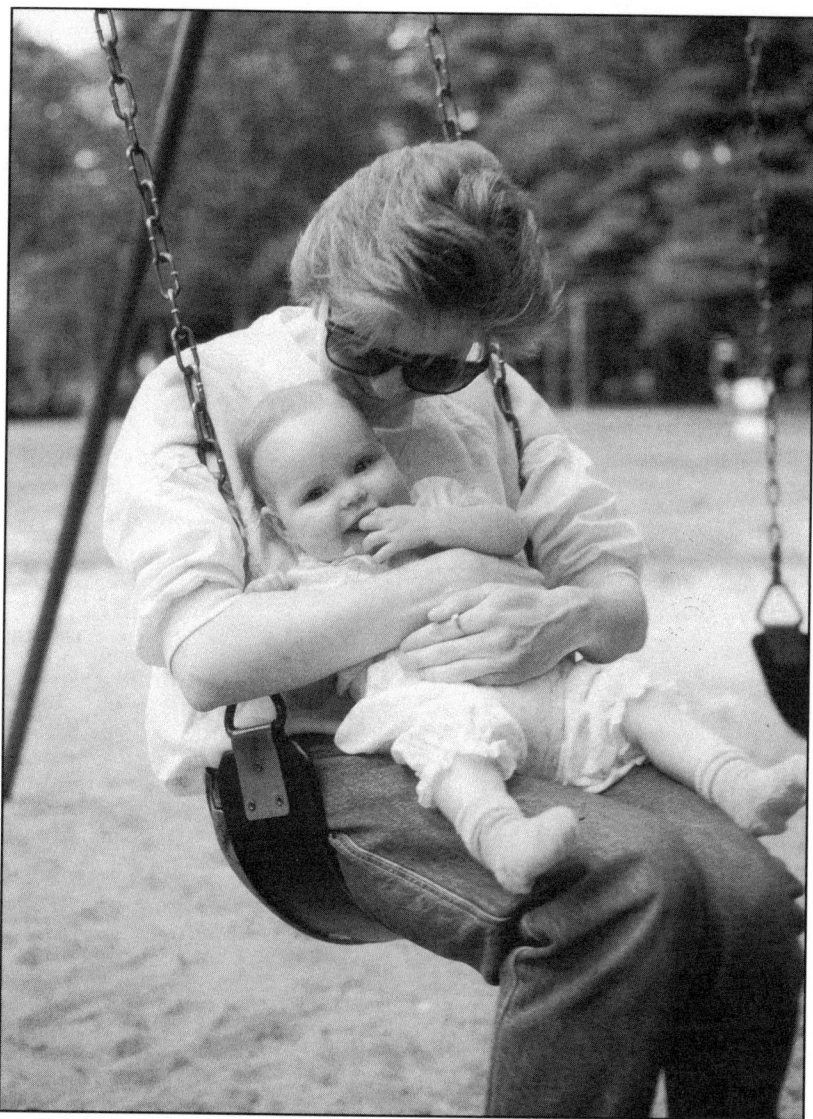

At the park, the swings are her greatest thrill.

makes silly faces for her. She giggles madly at any surprise tickle from me. We're finding out this month that Addie is a lot of fun to play with. Our time together goes by quickly. We can get so caught up playing on the floor in her bedroom, that when I turn around it's lunch time already and then time for her long nap. The days go by so quickly now. Sitting up has given her so much more flexibility and entertainment, and it has been reassuring for me as a mother. I worry. Oh, how I worry. (Though, I understand that I will do so for the rest of my life.) But for now my insecurities have abated. Adelyn has passed her first milestones, and while I can't take the credit, I can share in the victory. Today, sitting up. Tomorrow, the board room.

Dad's Thoughts

It's hard to believe Adelyn is eight months old. While it seems that it was just last week we brought her home for the first time, it feels like a lifetime since those first sleepless nights. Maybe it's because each day brings something new with her. Oh sure, the thrill of diapers has long since gone (if it was ever a "thrill"), and bathing and feeding her have become routine. But when I get Addie up from a nap, she still grins and wriggles in anticipation of being picked up—and that will never become routine for me. And the sound of her voice—I hope that never loses its magic, even when the language she uses is English.

Admittedly, it's pushing the point to try to be nostalgic after only eight months. But when I watch her my mind jumps back and forth between where she has been and where she is going. I don't want to lose this fascination—even when she is a teenager and driving Annie and me nuts with telephone calls and parties and, heaven forbid, boyfriends. Listen, I know it's unfair, but already I don't like teenage boys. It hasn't been that long since I was one—actually, it has been that long—but I still remember it very clearly. There is, I suppose, a sort of poetic justice in all of

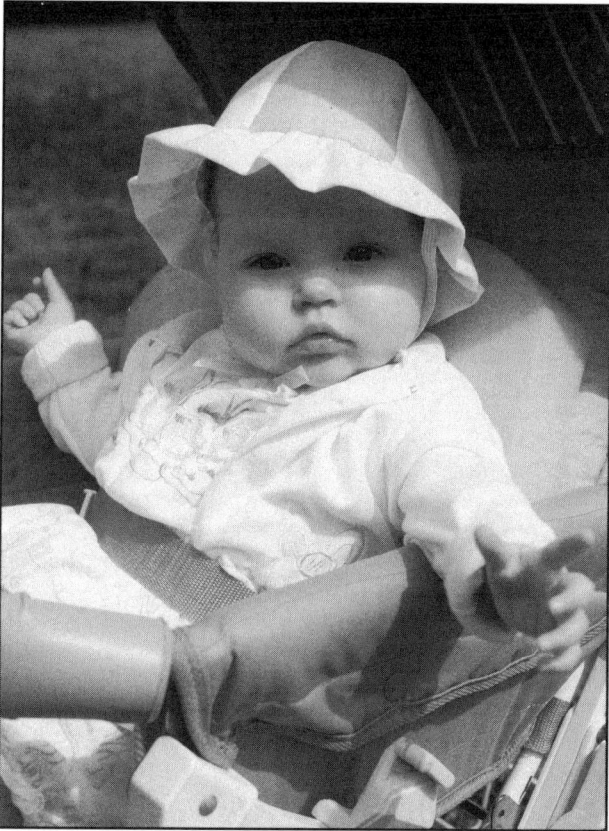

On her way to the park on a sunny afternoon.

this (when former teenagers become fathers), but it's difficult, now that I have a daughter, to appreciate the irony or
see the humor in the situation.

There is so much to learn between teething and the
teen years. And it's sort of an educational sprint. We'll have
to teach her everything we can before she turns fourteen,
when, in her eyes, Annie and I will become suddenly stupid. Sure, Ann and I will be able to resume her education
when she reaches twenty-one (according to Mark Twain),
but seven years in the abyss of ignorance is a very long time
to be away.

It's odd, I know, to be talking so much about Adelyn's
adolescence when she is just beginning her childhood de-

velopment. But I see her changing so rapidly, it's hard not to project. She sits with such confidence, I feel she is about to crawl any moment now. In the blink of an eye, she'll be walking. It seems that with each advance, the pace of change accelerates. The process of babyproofing will start very soon. As she begins to be mobile, table corners, light sockets, and stairs will be real hazards. As she gets older, becomes more autonomous, the threats she faces will be increasingly more complex, more insidious. Unfortunately, she will not always be aware of the dangers—not now, not fourteen years from now; and perhaps just as unfortunately, I will.

To be sure, if all parents had to worry about were table corners and teenage libido, life would be a breeze. But, it can be a nasty world; and I've thought long and hard about how to prepare her for it. But for now, I take great comfort in knowing my little girl is upstairs asleep in her crib.

Eighth Month—Pediatric Commentary by Dr. Marie Keith

The eighth month is the beginning of the Age of Mobility. The urge to get from here to there becomes an overriding passion. Babies are willing to work the entire day to master the possibilities of movement.

By now, the baby is quite adept at rolling over—from front to back and from back to front—and uses this interesting log roll to find her way to many unexpected places. But she soon finds that rolling is a difficult way to get where she wants to go. So

moving in a more directed way toward an appealing object becomes a new goal.

You'll remember that in the seventh month, many infants on their tummies usually push with their arms when motivated by some interesting object in their sight. But this pushing only moves babies away from the object. When they eventually realize they are moving in the wrong direction, most babies try pulling themselves with their arms and gradually inch forward.

This movement is actually very much like the movement of an inch worm—first the front part of the baby moves and then the back portion catches up, with the knees tucked in under the tummy and the buttocks raised up in the air. At this point, the arms are in position to pull forward again.

From this creeping maneuver, the more coordinated movements of crawling develop. The baby learns to keep the knees tucked under the tummy with the buttocks in the air and the arms bracing the upper chest off the floor. After practicing rocking in this position for some time, the baby then goes on to try to extend the right arm and the right knee, alternating with the left arm and left knee and voila! She is now crawling toward what she wants.

The other major development at this stage is to work on standing. At this age most babies have traded in those wobbly sea legs for sturdy legs that can straighten well and hold up the weight of the body. Parents will find that with very little support, babies will be able to maintain an upright standing posture for increasingly longer periods. They also enjoy bouncing in this position by bending their knees and springing back up again.

Through the course of the eighth month, many babies develop the ability to stand up while holding on. That is, when placed in a standing position with her hands grasping a firm support such as the edge of a chair or the rail of the crib or playpen, the baby can stand by herself. This is a very exciting moment for the infant and when you see the look in her eyes, you can tell she knows she's on to something.

Being placed standing is a great source of joy for the baby, but not nearly as wonderful as the next stage—pulling herself up to a standing position. Now any vertical surface such as the side rails of the crib, a wall, the legs of a chair or table or the softer legs of mom or dad become practice sites for the developmental stage called "pulling to stand."

Beginning in a crawl position, the baby will use her arms to pull up first to a kneeling posture. From the bent knee position, she brings one foot then the other to a flat position underneath her body and gradually pulls the upper body up with her arms. She is suddenly surprised and delighted to find herself in a standing position accomplished on her own!

With the ability to stand comes the greater likelihood of falls, so a few precautionary measures are in order. Babies often practice standing in their cribs, so it is clearly time to set the mattress at its lowest level and keep the side rails in the full, upright position so the baby doesn't stand and inadvertently fling herself out of the crib. Lots of large stuffed toys can serve as steps, putting the baby in a position to go over the rail, so avoid having these potential steps in the crib. Practice at standing should be done where falls can be softened, such as on carpeted floors, padded mats, or in the crib or playpen. Sharp edges or corners on low tables also pose a threat to a falling baby and should be padded.

Many babies enjoy a walker at this stage because they are happy in the upright position and like pushing with their legs for locomotion. Walkers are entertaining for babies as they allow the infant a means to get around. But the true skills needed for walking are developed more from the movements of crawling, standing, holding on, and the next stage, which is called "cruising," so babies should be given ample time to practice each of these.

A note of caution: Most walkers currently manufactured are made so they cannot collapse under the baby or tip over. Some, but not all, have built-in safety features to keep them from going down stairs. But the risks should be emphasized. The baby may fall down a step or stairway; she may move rather quickly to areas out of sight and into mischief; and she will have access to areas of danger that are somewhat higher than she could reach by crawling.

With so much energy devoted to developing locomotion skills, many babies seem to temporarily give up on vocalizing. Parents should not mistake this gap as a problem. When the time is right, your baby will devote more time to new efforts at vocalization.

Spurred on by a growing curiosity, the eight-month-old moves in many directions that can bring her to many potential dangers. So next month we'll consider aspects of childproofing that make a home a safe environment in which a baby can grow and develop. And we'll also talk about the next delightful stage of locomotion—cruising.

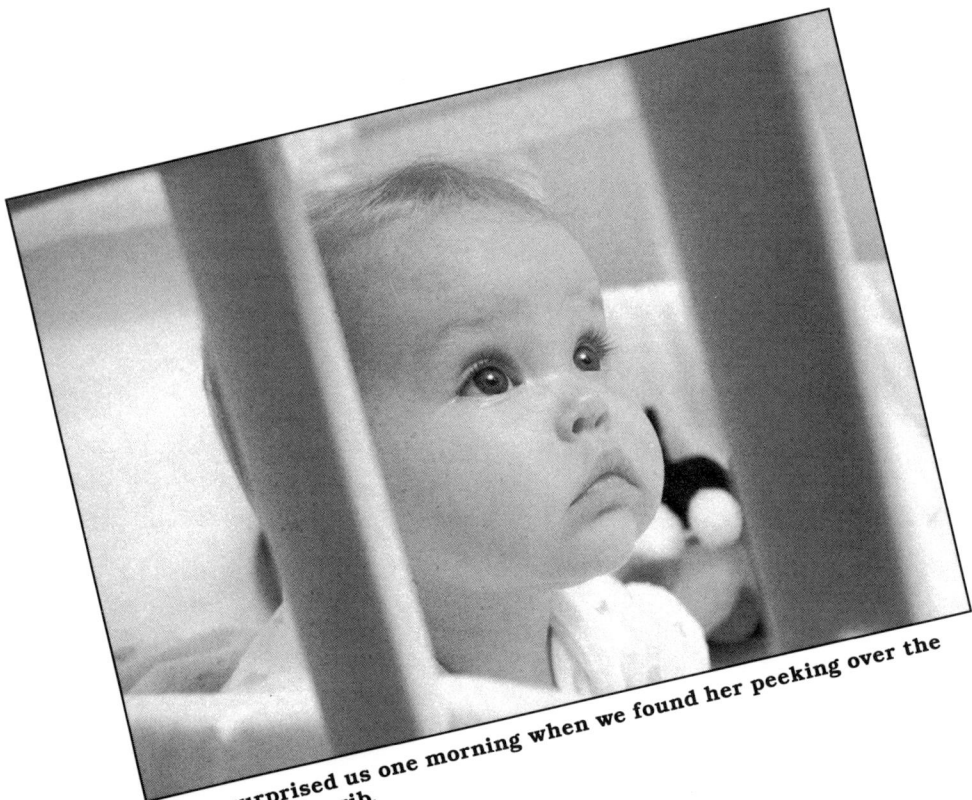

Adelyn surprised us one morning when we found her peeking over the bumpers of her crib.

Ninth Month

Mom's Thoughts

Nevin and I call it the "Call of the Crawl," otherwise known as the "Call of the Wild" (perhaps a more appropriate title).

While Adelyn started out the month riding high on her accomplishment of sitting up, by the middle of the month, she had become extremely frustrated in achieving her next milestone — crawling. Frequently, we've been awakened at about 5:00 A.M. to the sounds of Adelyn yelling in a rage. The first time I answered the yell and went into her room, I was surprised to see her peeking at me over the bumpers. This was a switch because she has always liked sleeping on her back. On awaking, she moves to her stomach and then begins the crawl scenario: First her head is up high with her legs flailing out from under her. Then she gets up on her knees, but at the same time, drops her head down flat on the mattress. Her behind moves back and forth, but there's no forward movement (yet). She screams her frustration with surprising ferocity. Nature is calling Adelyn, but she does not yet know how to respond.

As the month has progressed, Addie is now able to move one leg forward, but the other leg is not cooperating most of the time. So, for the most part, she moves backward, and she can cover a lot of distance in a surprisingly short time—when she wants to. Occasionally, Addie will move herself forward, but it's a very clumsy performance.

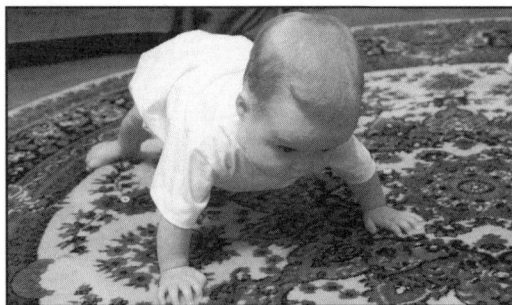

She's able to get herself up off the floor, but she hasn't figured out how to move forward yet. This shot is the prelude to one of her infamous swan dives.

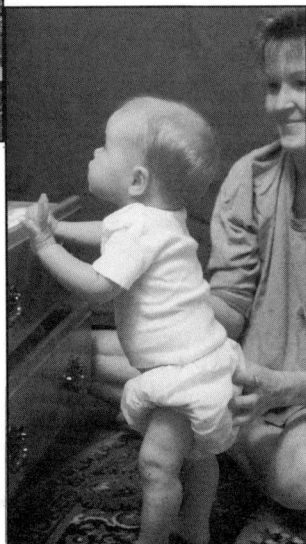

She needs a little help to get there, but Addie loves standing.

Her face pitches forward and she dives into the bed. I think one reason she doesn't like the floor is because it is not kind to her when she is practicing these swan dives.

But in her crib, Addie can move herself surprisingly well. She goes from one end to the other, from stomach to back, from one toy to another. I often wish that I had a video camera in her room to record what on earth she is doing up there as I hear a variety of sounds coming through her monitor. Bang, yell, coo, rustle, gurgle, shout. When I enter her room, she stops, and all attention is turned toward me. Of course, once she sees me, she wants out. Unfortunately, she is not yet as brave when she is out in the world as she is in her crib.

Adelyn also practices her crawling while breastfeeding, which is quite a feat! Her first feeding is taken between 6:00 and 6:30 A.M., and because she awakens so early, she gets fed in our bed. Lately, she has been wriggling from her side to her stomach as she is feeding and has been practicing crawling while eating. It becomes rather awkward for both of us, but I encourage her to crawl whenever I can. (Those days of holding that tiny little passive infant in my arms are *gone*.)

Adelyn also loves standing. She hasn't tried to pull her-self up yet, but I often stand her up now to put on her clothes, and she crows excitedly and gums my shoulders with her arms thrown around my neck. We often give each other "hugs" this way. The bureau drawers are fun to play in when I stand her up next to them. Addie plays with the clothes and pulls the handles up and down so that they make a funny noise.

Whether intentional or not (and probably not), Adelyn has begun sounding out familiar words. She said "Hi" clear as a bell one day after Nevin said it to her. She hasn't said it since that day, but it *was* an exciting moment. One day as I was putting her into her highchair, she said "Mama." She wasn't looking at me as she said this, but I was really thrilled to hear recognizable sounds at last. She recently said "Bobo" after I had been talking to her about our dog,

Beau, and it was the first time I really got the impression that she was imitating me. She is learning.

Her memory is also developing. Often when we read "Pat the Bunny" before bed, she will do all of the activities: Pat the bunny, play peekaboo with Paul, smell the flowers, touch Daddy's scratchy beard. At other times, when perhaps she is too tired to remember or just not interested, she will stare blankly at the pages.

Adelyn's snack time, which comes after her afternoon nap, has been a real learning experience for her over the past few months. While I used to worry about her choking on the teething cookie when it got very small, I have found that she can now gnaw and suck it to a very small size and then swallow it at the appropriate time. Adelyn has also recently learned to drink by herself from a cup. Earlier, she would drink so fast that most of the juice would be spit out, choked out, or poured down the front of her. (I used to dread snack time because of the mess that would be created.) With some guidance, however, she has gradually learned to drink a little bit slower, so she has time to swallow. She still frequently threatens to drop the cup over the side of her high chair, but often decides instead to bang it on the tray.

Addie enjoys banging anything she can get her hands on. She bangs two items together. She bangs things on furniture. She bangs things on the sides of her walker. She bangs things on me. While she had been doing this a little previously, she is now obsessed with hearing how things sound and her motions are repetitive. When I am fixing her meals, she's at it some more—bang, bang, bang, on the tray of her high chair.

We have a ritual when I'm preparing her meals. While I'm warming her food, I bring her a spoon so she can taste. (This started because she has always been impatient for her food.) She grins and grabs the spoon. When I first started doing this, she wouldn't take the spoon but expected me to feed it to her (my little princess). But I have been encouraging her and she has learned to take the spoon herself. So now I hear her banging the spoon after it has been licked clean.

While eating her meal recently, Addie picked up the extra spoon several times and started putting it into her mouth. The spoon, of course, had nothing on it and she eyed it rather disparagingly, but she kept doing it throughout the meal. I tried to indicate to her that she had to put it

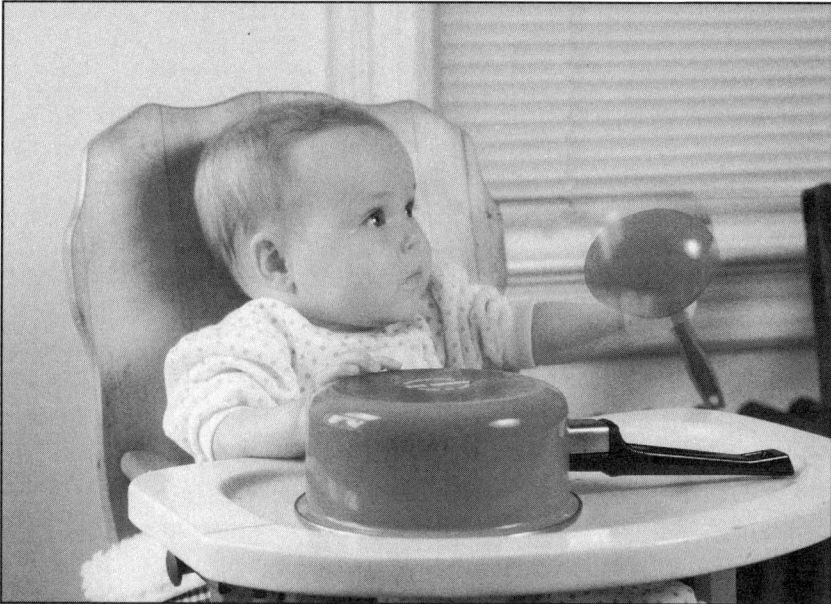

Addie enjoys banging anything she can get her hands on. She bangs things on furniture, she bangs things on her walker, she bangs things on me.

into the bowl first, but she didn't catch on. Sometimes I feel like I'm communicating with someone from another planet. How do you patiently teach the things that you've taken for granted all your life? I'm currently in the process of adjusting my mental faculties. We have a very long road ahead, and we have only just begun.

Dad's Thoughts

This morning, after breakfast, Adelyn and I discussed the letter "P." She sat on my lap facing me as I demonstrated the sound: "people," "puppies," "puff." "Puff" was her favorite. It aroused a belly laugh as she lunged toward me, burying her face in my shirt.

She loves to laugh. Irregular, staccato bursts: "Hee, hee (pause), hee (pause), hee, hee, hee, hmmmm." Although you cannot elicit laughter from her easily, when you do, it's worth the effort. Sometimes silliness will get her, sometimes it's just a simple word or phrase. More and more, though, Addie is finding her humor on her own. Certain things just strike her as being funny. In those moments, Annie and I realize our daughter is developing her own personality. And, I'm glad to see she has a good sense of humor. It will be a great asset.

Annie and I study her, trying to gauge her reactions. We want to be able to identify her personality tendencies. Researchers in child psychology have long argued the importance of heredity versus environment in the development of a child's personality. For many years, it was believed that environment played the most significant role. The current wisdom, however, asserts that heredity is a much more significant factor than previously thought. Meaning, I think, that a child's personality tendencies are determined genetically, *but* (and this is very important), the environment a child grows up in can minimize negative or undesirable traits and enhance or promote positive ones. Because of the importance of environment, parents must be perceptive. We must try to recognize early on the traits our children have brought with them into this world, and we must cultivate them judiciously.

Granted, certain responses, such as shyness, are exhibited by virtually all kids at some point or another. We have noticed that Addie becomes extremely frustrated when she tries to do something and can't. I think (I hope) that such reactions are less a sign of temperament and more a function of cognitive or physical development. I'm hoping that Addie's tendency to be easily frustrated is simply a result of her mind's ability to conceive an action that she hasn't the physical dexterity to execute, and that as she progresses, she will deal more effectively with initial failures. But knowing that a child's reactions aren't necessarily a sign of temperament only makes a parent's job harder. It is one more subtlety that must be taken into account.

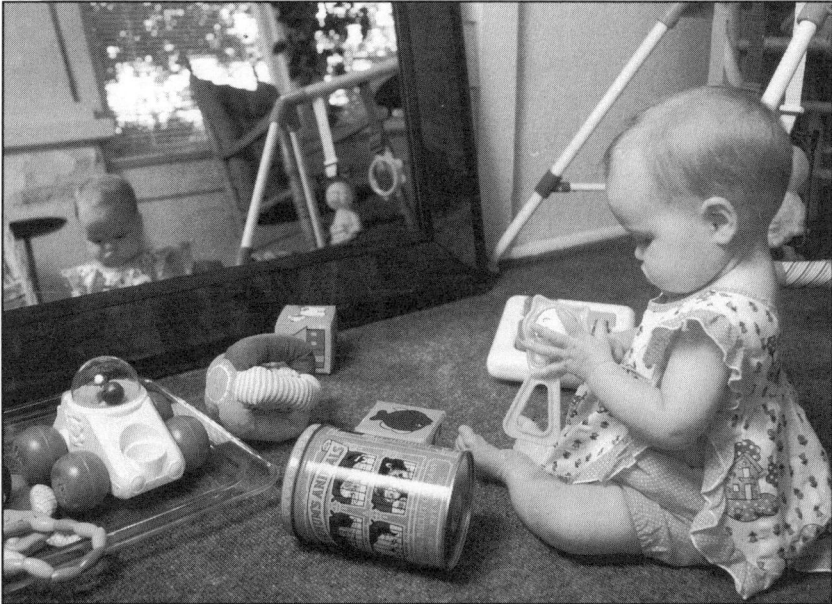

Sometimes she picks up a toy and studies it carefully, rolling it around in her hands over and over.

Addie also seems to balk at new things. Her first encounter with the walker is a perfect example. She was fine while it was stationary, but when she inadvertently moved backwards, she screamed. It wasn't long, though, before she became a pro in the walker. Her fear of new things bothers me a little. She will miss out on many successes if she's afraid to try something different. I hope Annie and I can stimulate her curiosity enough to overcome her fears.

One of the characteristics we're happy to see in her is what we perceive as a high concentration level. When she picks up a toy, particularly one that is new to her, she studies it carefully and with great intensity. She will not mouth it or bang it, simply study it, rolling it around in her hands over and over. Adelyn will not respond to noises, our voices, or anything when she is so absorbed. Also, she maintains this level of interest for a minute or two, which seems to me to be a fairly long time for a child that young. Ann also has that ability to focus her attention solely on the task at hand, and I have always been a little envious of this talent. I hope this aspect of her temperament is a permanent one.

Overall, Addie seems to be a basically happy child. She smiles easily, even at friends and family she has not met before or does not know well. And her smiles are very expressive. She has developed a sort of sly or mischievous smile— not a grin and not, I hope, a smirk. It comes when she looks at you out of the corner of her eye, her lips are pursed and just the ends of her mouth curl up. It is like a smile you'd see on a Dr. Seuss character and is, at least for me, extremely disarming.

I enjoy getting to know her immensely. Each day I learn more and more about her, and I like what I see.

Ninth Month—Pediatric Commentary by Dr. Marie Keith

In the ninth month, your baby is a vigorous, mobile and curious child. This combination leads the baby through a very significant phase of exploration marked by unimaginable mischief and the very real potential of serious harm through accidental injury. The words "baby-proofing" and "childproofing" were coined to help parents understand that the baby's home and environment must be a safe place in which possible hazards to the body are eliminated.

In the United States nearly 400 children under four years of age die every month because of accidents. Due to the enormity of the problem and the great personal tragedy a child's accidental injury or death is, this month's column is devoted entirely to safety issues.

Accidents often happen because parents are not aware of what their children can do. Babies learn fast and move quickly. In no time at all, an accident can occur. The American Academy of Pediatrics (AAP) has developed The Injury Prevention Program, called TIPP, to alert parents to dangers. Many of the following recommendations are presented in AAP literature and parents may wish to ask their pediatricians for these guidelines as they work on babyproofing their home.

Injuries from falls can happen to even younger infants who can wiggle and move, push against things with their feet and roll over. A fall from the height of a changing table can easily result in a fracture, concussion, blood clot around the brain, fractured clavicle, arm or serious neck injury, or lacerations. Never leave infants unattended on changing tables, beds, sofas, chairs, kitchen counters, or any other high places. Crib side rails should always be in the full upright position.

As the baby begins to crawl, move in a walker or cruise (walk holding on to furniture or walls), other dangers develop. Stairways should have protective gates both at the top and bottom. Windows should have guards, whether you think your child

can reach the windows or not. Falls down stairways or out of windows can lead to serious injuries to the head, back, or extremities and may cause death.

Sharp-edged furniture against which a child might fall should be padded or removed from the rooms in which babies play. A fall against a sharp-edged object can result in serious laceration or eye injury. Babies shouldn't play with sharp objects such as knives, forks, scissors, tools, pencils, lollipop or popsicle sticks, or breakable glass bottles, or ever be allowed to walk or crawl carrying them. A fall with such an item could result in severe laceration, eye injury, or injury to the mouth. If a child falls and hits her head, does not move her arms and legs normally, or has a laceration or eye injury, call your doctor immediately.

Burns are another source of accidental injury. Even a young infant can wave her fists and grab at things. Scald burns from hot coffee, tea, soup, or other hot foods can cause severe burns. Parents should never eat, drink, or carry anything hot near the baby. Stoves, ovens, wall or floor heaters, radiators, hot appliances, irons, and matches all become threats to the crawling or cruising infant. Babies and children do not know that these objects are hot and must be protected from them. The front burners on the stove, pot handles that extend away from the stove, and hot liquids, grease or food spilled on a baby all can cause serious burns. The best and safest place for your baby during food preparation is in the playpen or strapped in a high chair.

Electrical cords, wires, and outlets are another major source of burns or possibly electrocution. Protect electrical outlets not in use with plastic outlet covers. Electrical cords to appliances, lamps, etc., should not be on floor areas accessible to babies or dangling down walls within their reach.

Two other important ways to protect your baby against accidental burns are to equip your home with smoke alarms and reduce the temperature of the hot water to the range of 120-130°F. If your child does get burned, place the burned area in cold water immediately, cover the burn loosely with a bandage or clean cloth, and call your physician right away.

Choking and poisoning accidents are very real threats to a baby this age since she will put anything and everything into her mouth. Prevention of choking accidents begins with never leaving small objects in your baby's reach even for a moment. Balloons, marbles, small toy parts, and pen caps can be dangerous household items to the baby. Never feed her hard pieces of food or chunks that might lodge in her airway such as hot dogs, nuts, whole grapes, hard candy, raw carrots, apples, chunks of meat or peanut butter, popcorn, or raisins. Prepare food appropri-

ately for babies and be present while they are eating. Learn how to save a choking child through first aid classes or from your pediatrician.

Poisonings in babies occur from ingestion of household cleaning products and medications. All such items should be stored completely out of sight and reach of the baby. Safety latches on cupboard doors and drawers can help keep your baby away from potential dangers. If your baby does put something poisonous in her mouth, call your pediatrician or the Poison Control Center immediately. Have syrup of ipecac on hand to induce vomiting if you are instructed to do so.

The nine-month-old baby will love to play in water, so drowning accidents become a real danger. She can drown in even the most shallow water. Never leave a baby alone in or near a bathtub, pail of water, wading or swimming pool, or any other water, even for a moment.

The last danger to your baby, but certainly not the least, is car injuries. Automobile crashes are the greatest threat to your child's life and health. Car safety seats can prevent most auto injuries and deaths. By nine months, your baby, if over twenty pounds, will be ready for a forward-facing car seat. (Babies under twenty pounds must always face backwards.) Install your baby's car seat properly and use it according to instructions. Every time your child is in the car, she should be carefully buckled into place.

Always remember that pro-viding a safe environment for your child is a vital parental responsibility.

Seventh through Ninth Months— Child Development Commentary by Dr. Anita Hurtig

So much is happening in this seven to nine month period that Ann and Nevin are reeling. While we can at best hypothesize, based on careful observation, what was happening internally in the earlier four to six month period, Addie is now demonstrating actively, physically, and overtly her new found powers and her natural instinct to master, control, and expand her universe. This is the period of physical and psychological exploration and locomotion. And with locomotion and exploration comes distance.

Weaning is a first crucial step in the essential distancing that Ann and Addie are experimenting with. Ann recognizes that Addie sets her own pace in the process, gradually, but with a clear determination to move on to the next step, juice, cup, solids. Children who have difficulty with weaning may be demonstrating that they need more time with physical closeness and

quiet attention, that they are not ready to make the move toward increased separateness. Reluctance to be weaned may represent a mother's unwillingness to experience what Ann had earlier called a "letting go," because of ambivalence about giving up the closeness which infancy and breastfeeding offer. In these cases, it is wise for mothers to consider alternate ways of meeting their own needs, perhaps through renewed "talk"-time or playtime or feeding time, when intimacy can be shared in developmentally appropriate ways.

Ann and Nevin are again sensitively emphasizing a crucial element in their baby's development at this time—the role of play in encouraging physical as well as cognitive development. Play is, in many ways, the baby's work at this point of development. Piaget, Erikson, and other developmentalists have noted that play allows the infant to effectively explore, master, and control her environment. An infant who does not have the opportunity to bang, tear apart, put together, push, pull, create sound and make it disappear, feel hard and soft, and know what smells and what hurts, does not gain a sense of competence, does not learn. But as we read Ann's narrative, "Our time goes by so quickly—we can get so caught up playing on the floor of her bedroom . . .," we realize that Addie's environment is a very special and unique one.

In many of the families we meet and work with, these long and special moments are not present. In families with only one parent, usually a mother who finds she must be out of the house in order to work, leaving her baby with uncertain caretakers, babies do not necessarily have these necessary experiences of stimulation. Statistics indicate that even in two-parent families more mothers of infants are working than remaining at home. There is no clear evidence that babies of working mothers are at greater risk for developmental problems. But research does clearly indicate that babies who are not given consistent and frequent stimulation—who do not experience positive interactions—are less likely to receive these essential attentions in early childhood and are more vulnerable to reduced cognitive functioning and to social withdrawal or acting out. Ann and Nevin's unique status as at-home workers allows them to "care" for their baby *and* accomplish

their essential adult social/economic roles. The challenge to less fortunate families is one which our society has not yet approached with clear social policy commitments. It is a problem that presents a hazard for babies not as well situated as Addie.

Addie has other advantages which enrich her development in these middle months of her first year. In addition, and related to exploration and locomotion, this is a period of complex interpersonal growth, as Addie begins to realize that she not only has a mind of her own, but that others can share her mind with her. Thus, her intentions ("give me my cup" or "give me my juice") or her pleasures (touching Daddy's beard, playing peekaboo with Momma) are shared, responded to, and encouraged. Addie checks to make sure both parents and even Grandpa are sharing her world. The opportunity to share is basic to the development of the capacity for empathy. Parents who, like Ann and Nevin, enjoy "getting to know" their infant are helping her to build the capacity for enjoying others.

Nevin touches on an issue that is sensitive for all parents. How much responsibility must a parent(s) take for the development of the child's personality? We are all familiar with the kind of mother-bashing that has left mothers feeling guilt-ridden if their baby or child or adolescent isn't perfectly adjusted, whatever that may be. Nevin comes out on the side of a balance between heredity and environment, recognizing that there are certain temperamental features which may show up early (Addie's shyness and perseverance) but which get modified, positively or negatively, by early forces and interactions. This is a safe and calming position for a parent to take, and probably the most realistic one as well. It allows for the child's natural temperament to be expressed, but recognizes that rearing can inhibit or encourage a baby's natural instincts to master and control in a safe and protective environment. Specifically, Nevin's concerns over Addie's hesitation with new experiences is a natural one, particularly for a father whose approach is so assertive. But Addie's behavior is healthy and adaptive. She is ready to learn and it is the parents' role to stimulate and encourage. When Addie feels overwhelmed by the demands of the task, Ann and Nevin are there to support and assist. Their positive and patient approach is one which allows Addie to use her newfound skills over and over in increasingly complex ways to meet the challenge and move on to the next one.

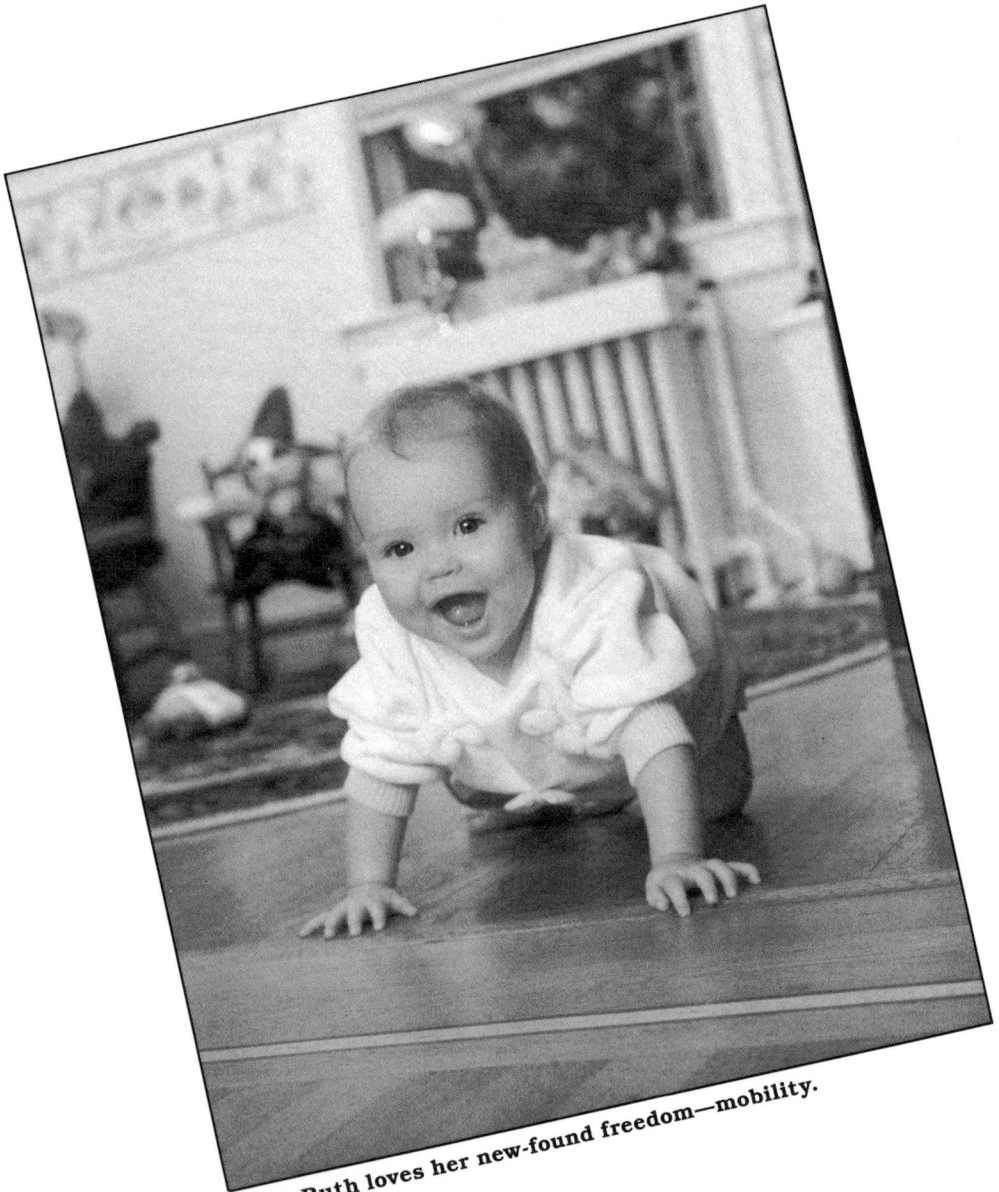

Addie Ruth loves her new-found freedom—mobility.

Tenth Month

Mom's Thoughts

Look out world, Adelyn Ruth Kishbaugh is mobile. Within days of her nine-month birthday, Addie coordinated her movements in the appropriate direction, and by month's end, she had become an accomplished crawler. Other achievements followed rapidly: She can get herself in a sitting position, go up the first three steps of our staircase to the landing, pull herself up in her crib and on the sofa, and she can take a few steps while standing. Addie has been very busy this month practicing all of her new movements. I've been very, very busy this month following Addie (and cleaning the floors). Luckily, I had been expecting this to happen and had done most of the babyproofing, but I still keep a watchful eye on her to see what I may have over-looked and to keep her from being too brave. (And to think that I was worried about her progress not so long ago!)

Addie has been a delight to watch as she masters each task she sets her mind to. Every day has added something new to her repertoire. It seems odd to think that last month we were thrilled when she peeked her head over the bumpers. Imagine our joy when we went to get her after her nap and saw her standing at the crib railing, grinning from ear to ear. My primary function now is serving as Adelyn's jungle gym. When I join her on the floor, she gets this par-ticular gleam in her eye and guns for me. Her hands clutch and crawl her way up my body until she is standing tall be-side me excitedly dancing back and forth on her tiptoes.

To show her pleasure at this accomplishment and for my cooperation, Addie gives me what used to be a kiss, but now has become a bite. It used to be cute when she gum-med my shoulder, but she is having trouble learning to withhold the teeth when she "kisses" me now. All in good time, but I do hope it is soon!

Yes, Adelyn now has six teeth (and I understand that this is all she will get for a while). We recently made the switch to junior foods to give her practice chewing. I found that frequently as she was motoring around the house, I would hear an unusual sound accompanying her. It was the sound of her teeth chewing. That's when I knew strained foods were no longer necessary for this child. She's enjoying the tiny bits of food and having fun picking up the noodles in the junior dinners.

Addie will use a spoon when the mood hits her, and she does it surprisingly well. I show great enthusiasm, despite the fact that often some food has dribbled down the side of the high chair and landed on the dog's ear. I bought her a short spoon that is good for beginners, and while she is eat-

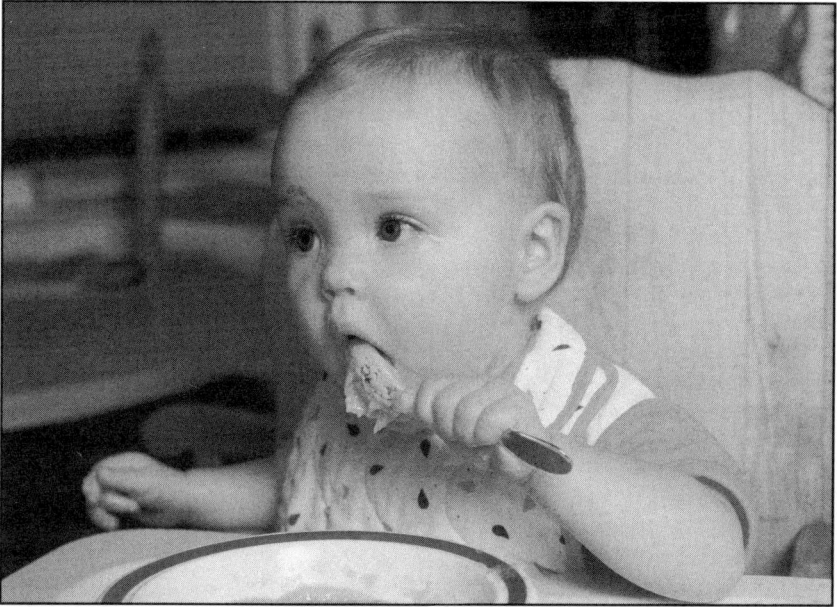

Adelyn uses a spoon surprisingly well. Although this picture doesn't show the previous spoonful that landed on the dog's head.

ing, I leave it in her fruit for those times when the spirit moves her. (I'm hoping that fruit, which she loves, will give her an incentive. Funny, the tricks you make up as childrearing progresses.)

To give her practice, I also leave a little bit of food on her plate, then busy myself with other things in the kitchen because I know she will feed herself if left to her own devices. (When I'm sitting in front of her, Addie tends to demand that I do it for her.) It takes all my courage to move away because I know what will result. I tell myself she needs to learn this; therefore, I need to let her learn it. Newspapers surrounding the high chair do help the cleanup detail. And, of course, the dogs do their part.

Adelyn has also been weaning herself from breastmilk this month and is down to one breastfeeding in the morning. Because my doctor recommends starting milk at one year of age because of the possibility of allergies (I have a milk allergy), Adelyn is drinking formula now. The weaning was gradual, and with the addition of those new teeth, I am not particularly saddened at this turn of events. Adelyn has been biting a lot lately, and while I have tried to be firm with her and very patient, it has been putting a strain on our relationship. I am pleased that I stuck with it this long, but I am relieved that we have moved apart in a natural manner because I had been considering weaning her myself. We still enjoy our time in the morning, but I can see that the end is near on that feeding also.

All was well at Adelyn's nine-month check-up this month. She is progressing well, albeit slowly, and the doctor was pleased to hear about her new developments. On seeing Adelyn this time, he remarked in surprise, "She *really* looks like Nevin." Adelyn was happy playing with his watch and stethoscope while we talked, and as no shots were given this time, she left with a smile on her face.

An interesting change has occurred in Adelyn this month. She has become a show-off when we are out. Addie used to stare at everyone with great intensity, giving smiles only on rare occasions, but at the doctor's office, she actually yelled at the women across the aisle to get their attention. When she had their attention, Addie beamed broadly and babbled away in response to their questions to her. Grandma Sandt, my mother, is particularly thrilled with this new development because she has always tried so hard to coax smiles from her latest grandchild. Not anymore. Adelyn needs no coaxing and beams broadly on first seeing her. Recently, we were watching a videotape of a family reunion, and when Adelyn heard her grandmother's voice, she swiveled around from what she was doing on the floor and watched the screen intensely.

While Adelyn has come out of her shell, true to what I've read, she has developed some separation anxiety toward me with the development of her increasing mobility. At times, she gets very upset when I leave a room or leave her sight, and she has difficulty going to sleep at night despite our nightly rituals. I'm trying to reassure her with my voice, and we are trying different strategies at night, but it is becoming increasingly frustrating for all of us. As with other problems, we know it's only a matter of time before we hit upon the right solution or she heads into another phase.

As Dr. Keith predicted, Addie's daily babbling has slowed with the development of her mobility. She says "momma" frequently, and, at times, I know she means me, but sometimes she says it as if she's just practicing the sound. She also says "baba" a lot, but she uses it for different items—the dog, her toy rings, the ball. However, a couple of incidents have occurred that let us know her comprehension is improving. I have played "Where is your _____?" with her a few times, and one particular time she was very responsive and went to look for the things I requested—Big Bird, her telephone, and the ball. At other times, she'll look for one item or none. On another occasion, her dad and I were having a "discussion," and she kept shouting louder and louder until we had to stop what we were doing and pay attention to her contribution.

I've also noticed that Addie really enjoys nursery rhymes now. I frequently recite them to distract her while I'm changing her diaper—Addie has no time for diapering now. (I'm so afraid that I'll accidentally stick her with a pin one of these days!) And occasionally, when she is very tired, she will lie in my arms with a toy and listen to my whole repertoire while I bounce her in time with the rhythm. It's also useful for word association when I use her Mother Goose book.

Addie's emerging abilities have caused me some concern. Two incidents occurred on the same day: first, Addie attempted to catapult herself off of the bed toward the phone on the nightstand. I caught her in midair. Later I returned to her room after dumping her diaper and found that she had one of the extra diaper pins in her hand. I was shaken. That night I dreamt that she fell down the stairs. My mother reminds me of the time that she found my sister sitting in the window of their third-floor apartment and leaning on a loose screen. She still remembers her dreams that night. You can't be too careful. According to Mom, these dreams will continue throughout Addie's childhood and beyond. But that's all they are—dreams. In a way, the dreams serve as an extra caution. With a lot of forethought and knowledge, and careful planning and teaching, we can protect her from many things and teach her to protect herself. We have been charged with a formidable responsibility.

Dad's Thoughts

Yes, it finally happened—Adelyn is mobile—and Annie and I are burning up a significant number of calories following her around. It happened one morning after breakfast. Addie and I were playing on the floor. She had her eye on a toy that was far out of her reach. I moved it a little closer to entice her—but still a full body-length away. She was already on her hands and knees, rocking back and forth—which was something she had learned several weeks before. She looked at the toy on the floor, grinned, and stumbled forward. The approach was not graceful, but she and I were quite thrilled. It was no less momentous an occasion than Greg LeMond's first Tour de France triumph, no less exciting than Franco Harris' "immaculate reception."

But this was no spontaneous accomplishment. She had been in training for this for weeks—months really. It began by simply trying to get her to accept being on her stomach. She resisted, of course, the way she has resisted most changes.

Not long after she accepted being on her belly, she began to push herself up with her arms, her legs still flat against the floor. This strengthened her arms and back, but forced her body backwards. She soon started to push up with her legs, her butt to the sky, forming a sort of inverted "V." It got her up in the air, but she still couldn't go anywhere.

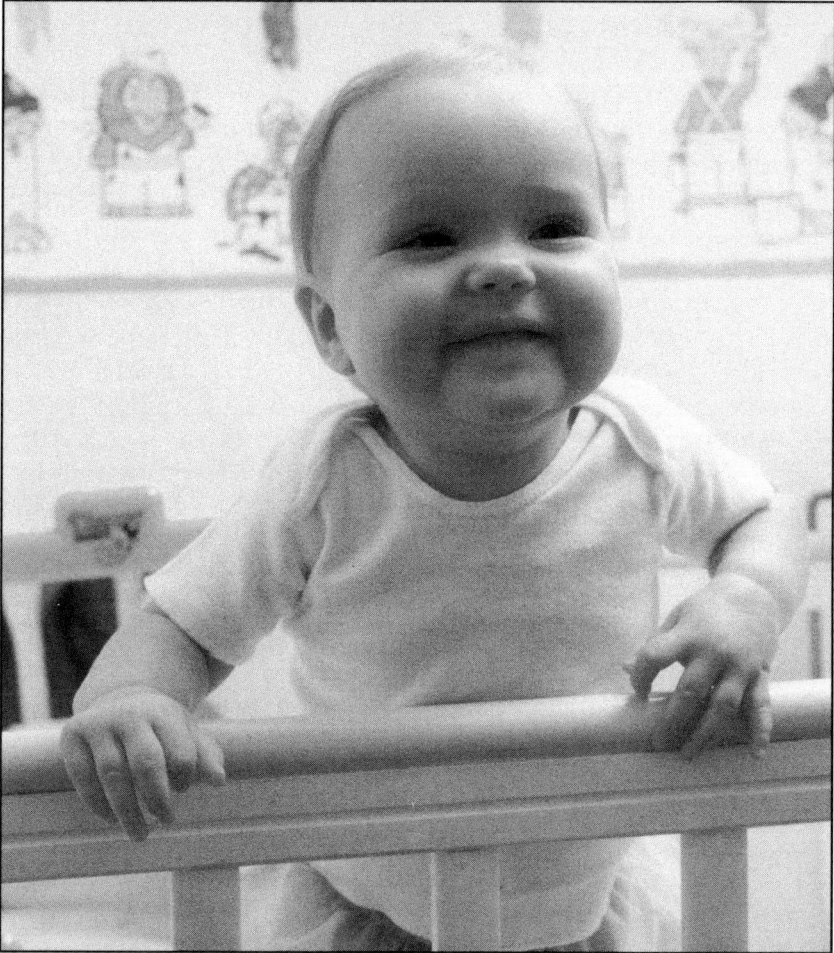

Only a month ago, we were thrilled to find Addie Ruth peeking over her crib bumpers—now look at her. She's pretty proud of herself, too.

The next step in the evolution of the crawl was for Adelyn to bring her knees up underneath her—to support her weight on her hands and knees. Once she accomplished this, we knew she could crawl at any time. We watched her expectantly, encouraging and enticing her with toys placed beyond her reach. She would lunge for them, but invariably she'd end up flat on her stomach. Although it took her a couple of weeks to put all the movements together, the practice was worth it.

As she practiced crawling after that eventful morning, I noticed that she had developed an unusual variation of the standard hand-knee, hand-knee crawl. Adelyn would stick her left leg out to the side and push off the floor with either foot instead of her knee. We guessed that she was either trying to save wear and tear on her knee, or that she was simply trying to stand up. In fact, after only a few days of crawling, she did pull herself up into a standing position—and she was quite proud of herself for doing so. (She still uses that sidewinder crawl—but only occasionally.)

From crawling came standing, and from standing came climbing. We have an enclosed front porch which has become Adelyn's primary playground. It held her toys, her highchair, gave her plenty of room to roam, and was safe because she couldn't negotiate the step that led into the living room. At least we thought she couldn't. One morning, after breakfast (did you notice that so many things happen in our house after breakfast?) I was taking her dishes out to the kitchen when I heard a noise behind me. I turned to find Adelyn pushing herself up on the step into the living room. Forget the dishes, this was a very precarious place for her to be. In the three seconds it took me to get to her, she was already over that hurdle and heading toward one of the dogs when she realized what she had done. She spun around, sat down, and grinned at me. There's no stopping her now. If we put her on the floor of the porch, we might as well start walking toward that step—that's where she's headed. She loves to climb, and we let her as long as we're around. If we're going to leave her alone for anytime at all, the gate must go up.

With all this exercise, you'd think Addie would be sleeping like a rock. Not quite. Actually, she does sleep soundly, but only because it's taken an hour and a half to put her down. She does not "go gentle into that good night," she screams bloody murder instead. All of this is quite strange to us. We've been sort of spoiled. Up until now, there's been no problem getting her to sleep—except for the occasional teething or other specific problem. So when her protests first started (at my father's one night), teething and/or gas were the first culprits that came to mind. Yet, we noticed, or rather Ann did, that Adelyn's cries were not those of pain, but of terror.

Having read that sleep disturbances were common around nine months, we concluded that all this crying was an extension of the separation anxiety she had been exhibiting lately. We were sure of this when she calmed down when Annie went to her. But we did not want to give in so easily. We thought that letting her cry would be the best thing for everyone in the long run. Unfortunately, her cries only became more desperate, and after twenty or thirty minutes, we had to intervene.

Through trial and error, we came up with something of a solution. We take more time than usual putting her to bed. It is now a very slow process that gradually acquaints Addie with the fact that we are going to leave her. Ann reads several books to her, sings quietly, rocks her slowly while standing before her crib, and when she does put Addie down, she stays in her room or within shouting distance to soothe her as necessary. Addie still manages to leap to her feet a few times before we are completely successful. But at this point, we've reached a truce, albeit a tenuous one.

I would have to say that this is the single most frustrating problem we've encountered so far. Her screams were at once both heart-wrenching and maddening. We knew there was nothing wrong, but we were powerless to convince her of that. Your initial reaction is to comfort her—to rock her and sing her to sleep—but after twenty minutes with a child screaming in your ear, all you want to do is disappear. And believe me, the guilt associated with that feeling is quite powerful. But more compelling than that is the realization that your child fears, above all else, that you will desert her—that she will be alone forever. I could never, ever let her believe that.

Tenth Month—Pediatric Commentary by Dr. Marie Keith

In Addie Ruth, as in other children at about ten months of age, we start to see the beginnings of separation combining with an emerging sense of self.

"Look out world, here I come." This paraphrase of her mother's opening statement is definitely how Addie Ruth views her life as a baby who is now ten months old and beginning to make her presence known.

Something dramatically different, new, and fascinating develops in the psyche of children this age as they begin to see themselves as their own person. Although Addie has displayed her personality, temperament, and social interaction from an early age, we begin to sense that in some way she has now integrated all of these features and begun to internalize them into a sense of her own identity. What follows is an understanding, at a very tender level, that she exists as a separate being, as Addie Ruth Kishbaugh.

In all that Ann and Nevin describe of Addie's new accomplishments, we see her making inroads toward the development of independence. Foremost is her mobility. After weeks and months of practice, Addie has learned to move by crawling, climbing, or cruising, and now she can move toward a desired object. It is this exact movement toward something new that also

takes her away from the familiar and known. She is now able to distance herself from the safe arms of her mother or father and know that she is separated.

A developing sense of self is also evident during feeding time in babies Addie's age. Younger infants are fed passively; they open their mouths and receive the food. But ten-month-old babies become active participants in feeding—and often demand to "do it themselves." Their pincer grasp usually is quite controlled by now and the babies enjoy finger foods they can pick up and put in their mouths. These babies also get better at manipulating a spoon. As Ann describes, Addie very often aims right to her mouth (although, as pointed out, there is also a lot of flying food.)

Addie will also feed herself when left to her own devices—a very independent act.

Another clear example of her development of self is her vocalizations for social interaction. Addie, as an individual, yelled to some women who were complete strangers in order to focus their attention on herself. And when her parents were trying to have a discussion, she wanted her contribution to the discussion to be noted. Although unable to speak in words, she is now aware that her utterances provoke a clear response from others. She independently chooses to make sounds as a participant in the social milieu.

A realization has begun to dawn on her, in a very primitive form, that she is no longer just an extension of her mother or father but truly her own being. Addie Ruth is ready to meet the world as herself. This is an exciting moment for her but it's also frightening, so we see the emergence in Addie of the first stage of separation anxiety.

The paradox of babies at this age is that at the same time there is movement toward independent behavior, there is an intense need to be close. Babies tread a very fragile line between being their own person and being a part of their parents. This dilemma produces a fair amount of anxiety especially in the arena of sleep problems.

It is not at all unusual for babies at this juncture to have difficulty drifting off to sleep. The need to hold on to someone who is close and the fear of letting go into the realm of sleep are very potent forces. As Ann and Nevin have discovered, Addie needs a lot more reassurance of their presence in her life now than she did before.

And, as her parents have astutely observed, this is a developmental phase which Addie will pass through. In time, as she begins to comprehend what is happening—even though only at an infant level of understanding—she will know that although she is herself and very much her own being, her parents are always right there beside her.

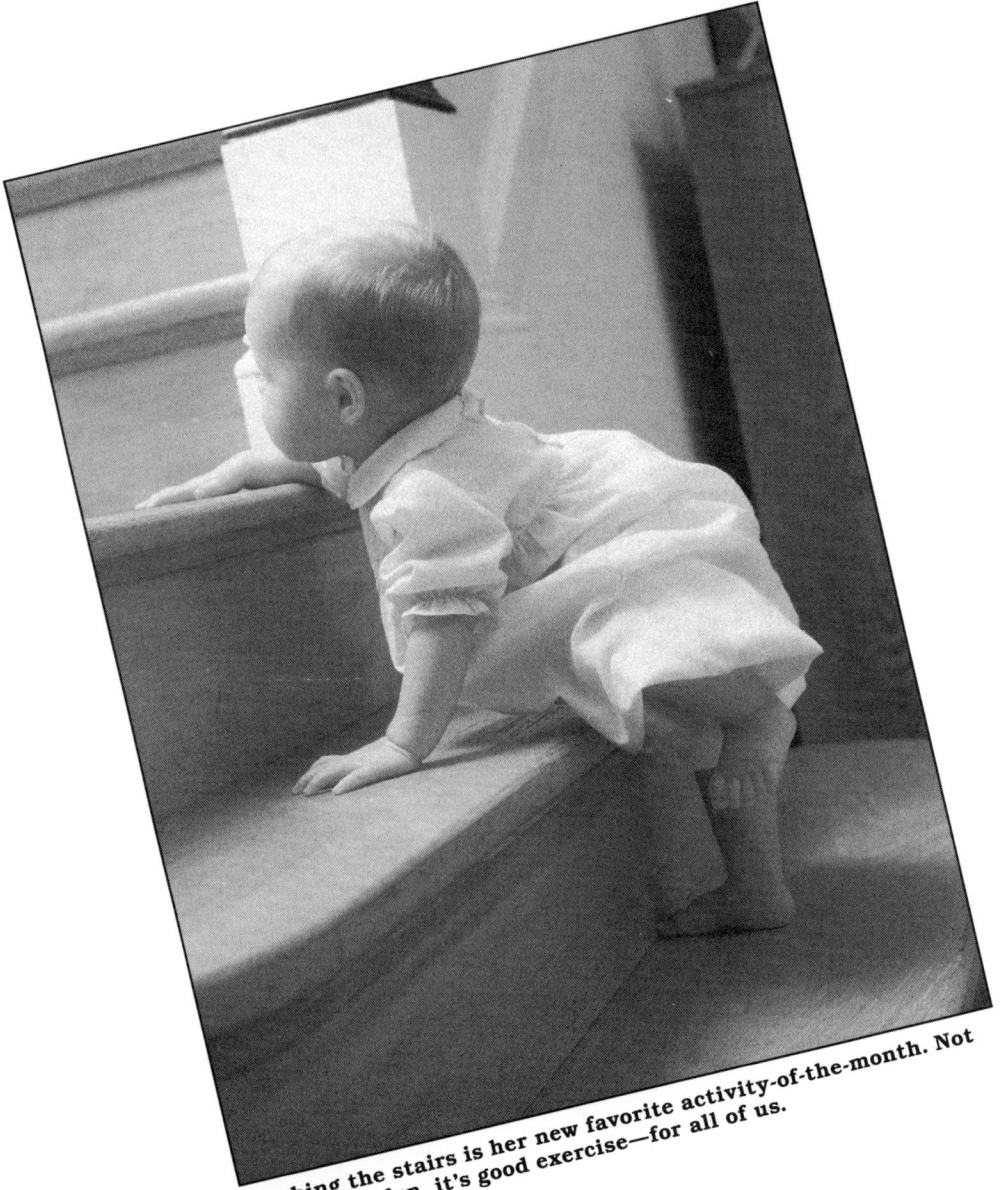

Climbing the stairs is her new favorite activity-of-the-month. Not only is this fun, it's good exercise—for all of us.

Eleventh Month

Mom's Thoughts

These are the times that try mother's (and father's) souls. Sleeping problems continued as we passed Addie's ten-month birthday. Addie simply did not want to sleep anymore. She was miserable from lack of sleep. We were miserable from lack of sleep. We comforted. We cajoled. We commanded. We sat in agony outside of her bedroom door listening to the screaming.

My sister Sue stressed that we must be consistent in whatever we chose to do. But one of the problems might have been that Nevin and I had different ideas about how things should be handled. So we discussed the exact plan of action. We mapped our routine down to the exact seconds we would stay with her before leaving her bedroom and, if necessary, go back in to comfort her further. Most importantly, we were consistent in what we did.

After five days, a miracle happened. I left her bedroom and all was silent. Oh, the sweet sounds of silence. We sat in the living room in disbelief. Dare we hope that we had crossed the threshold? Addie returned to her two-nap-a-day schedule the next day. She went quietly to sleep the next night. All was well. The house breathed a sigh of relief.

During the day, Addie babbles constantly. Her current favorite sound is "mamama," which she repeats throughout the day, so much so that it has become like background music. I have also heard "dada" and sometimes she will say "anana," which I think means banana, but the "m" sound is the hands-on favorite this month. When we went to the store recently, I heard "mamama" being said in a very different tone. When I turned, I saw it was a little boy using the exact sound in the same manner as Addie. I have read that if I went to China, I would also hear the same sound. Addie does use "mamama" in distress and appears to know that I will come in response to it. I'll be thrilled when I'm certain she means me—and won't it be nice when "I love you" and a hug are thrown in too!

Addie has not made as many leaps in her physical abilities this month as in previous months, but a few of her new activities are noteworthy. She can scale the entire staircase (eighteen steps) in a very few minutes. She and I do this at least five times a day. While at times it can be very tiresome for me to do this over and over, its's excellent for Addie. It strengthens her legs for standing and, someday, walking (and is also very good for me). Next month we'll concentrate on learning how to back down the steps.

Addie can also lower herself to the floor from a standing position. At first she would come crashing to the floor (it's nice that her diapers provide such padding) with arms flying. By the end of the month, she had perfected the movement so that she lowered herself very slowly, even gracefully, using her hands for balance. She repeats this exercise over and over.

Another milestone was passed this month—Addie had her first childhood illness. When I got her out of her crib one day after her nap, I could feel that she was very hot. Her temperature was 103°F. Addie was glassy-eyed but seemed rather calm. I, however, was panicked and raced for the phone with my Dr. Spock book in hand. The doctor saw us right away but he could detect no clear illness. He suggested that I stop giving her breastmilk/formula and solid food and switch to Pedialyte while her fever was high for a day or two, and that I give her Infant's Tylenol to help bring the fever down. At this point, she was becoming very irritable, and for the next few days until her fever subsided, she slept a great deal and was cranky when awake.

When the fever finally ended and she appeared normal, I noticed a rash much like measles starting to spread up her legs and torso. I again ran for the phone. Of course, it was Saturday afternoon and doctors' hours had already ended. The doctor on call advised us to come in right away, and within minutes, he had diagnosed her as having roseola infantum or "baby measles." He prescribed an antibiotic and told me not to worry because the rash meant the disease was in its last stage. Addie was calm and appeared to be fine. The rash didn't affect her in the least. It continued to spread for another day and then vanished as quickly as it had come. Phew! One illness down, about fifty more to go.

In the past few months, I've noticed that my role as a mother is changing. At first I was primarily Addie's caretaker—feed, burp, change, amuse, feed, burp, etc. Now I am moving into the role of being Addie's playmate and teacher. It seemed to happen gradually. At first you do all the things the books tell you to do. Talk to them, sing to them, show them things, demonstrate for them. But you don't really think that you are getting through.

When Addie waved "Hi" recently to her grandfather for the first time, I looked at her in wonder. We are getting through! Think of all the things I can tell her and show her and teach her. It hit me like a truck. Later, I was in the kitchen doing dishes with one eye on Addie. She, of course, headed for the dogs' water bowl. I have repeatedly told her "No" when she goes to play in it. Within inches of the bowl, she stopped, turned to look up at me, gave me a sly grin, and veered off in another direction. I bet Addie is also thinking of all of the things she can teach me!

My oldest sister Ruth recently came to visit. Since she lives quite a distance, she hasn't been to our house since Christmas. After walking in the door and exchanging greetings, she said, "Yep, you can tell a child lives in this house now. Houses always look a lot different."

Yes, the old homestead has changed quite a bit. Various toys are piled in corners or strewn about depending on what time of day it is. There are gates to climb over or remove as needed. Some furniture has disappeared to make play areas. There is a playpen in the corner now and a high chair with bibs piled high in the corner. Yep, things have certainly changed.

Addie's room was recently rearranged to give her a larger playing area. I practically emptied the room out except for her crib and dressers, and we babyproofed the room thoroughly. She likes playing there a lot. Her favorite activity for the past few weeks has been to empty her bookshelf of all of her books. She looks over the books even as she is discarding them over her shoulder. Sometimes she stops to examine a favorite. She gnaws at them and tries to turn the pages. She piles them up. She steps over them. They're fun to slide on. Even better to slide on is Beau, who often sprawls out on the floor. (It is a good thing that he is so gentle and easy-going.)

I am constantly recirculating toys. Different ones are put away each day or put in another room. (Each room has an area with at least a few toys in it.) One or two different toys are placed in her crib each day to keep her busy for a few more minutes on those mornings when she decides to begin her day at 5:00 A.M. My sisters have very generously passed on their children's old toys, which has been a god-

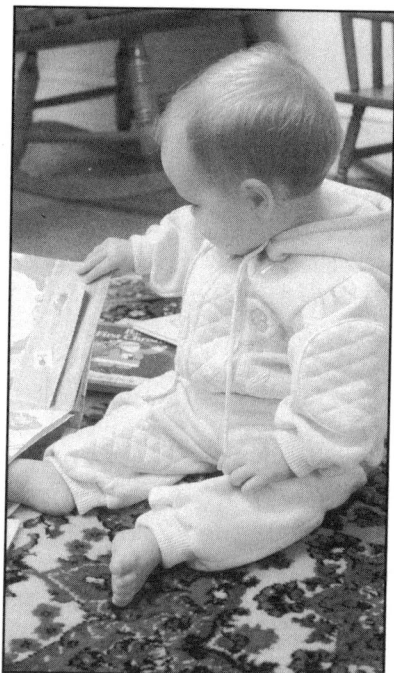

Adelyn loves books. She sorts through her whole collection, stopping only to examine a favorite.

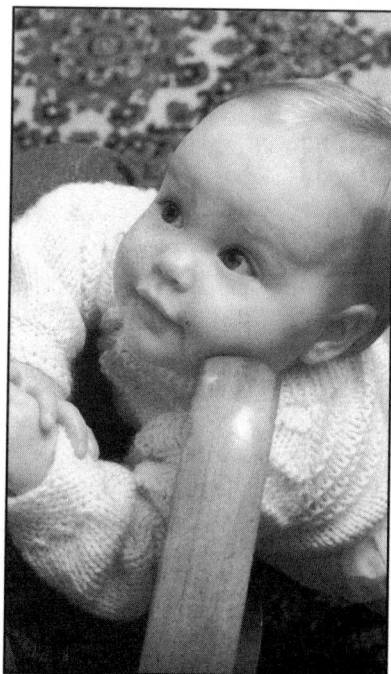

When Addie has found one she likes, we read it to her.

send to our budget, but she still appears to be insatiable for that "something new" to pique her interest for more than a few minutes.

I examine every container that I throw out for Addie potential. Squirt bottles are rinsed out thoroughly for floating toys. Aluminum pie plates make a neat noise. Oatmeal containers filled with an old rattle make a neat toy to crawl with and push. All the empty containers do nicely to fill in gaps, and it's amazing how many household items can also be drafted for use. Of course, I examine them carefully for anything with potential danger.

A very favorite toy is still the car keys, but I save this as a very special treat as needed. Addie can sit on the wooden floor for half an hour with the ring of keys, dropping it again and again, pushing it around and around. A shoebox filled with scarves and some plastic lids is fun to play in while I'm getting dressed to go somewhere. Another favorite is bangle bracelets. I usually wear them if we're going someplace to visit where I don't think there will be toys so she can keep herself out of mischief for a little while.

Addie and I are learning to play together. For the most part, I observe, trying not to interfere with her efforts. She likes me around and I like being around. When she accomplishes something new, she looks over and grins. When she is on uncertain territory, she looks back for fortitude. Occasionally, I'll show her how to operate a toy, but I've found that it is better if she finds things out on her own. Sometimes we'll romp on the bed or look out the window together at the passing traffic. Our favorite game, however, is "I'm gonna get you." As you probably guessed, I crawl around on the floor after her repeating this phrase in menacing tones. Addie squeals in delight as she "runs" for cover.

My father called the other day after he had been away on a trip. He had stayed at the home of a couple with a child who was Adelyn's age and awakened in the morning to the merry sound of happy singing in the kitchen below. Daniel, the little boy, was actively participating in the singing with his mother and father, and my father was taken with the delightful scene. He asked the mother for the name of the tape. We both looked for it and came up with it a few days later. The tape, "Morning Magic" by Joanie Bartels (Discovery Music), is wonderful.

As Nevin has noted, I'm not really a morning person. After I stumble sleepily down the stairs with Adelyn in my arms, I now head right for the tape deck and pop in this tape. I put Adelyn in the playpen while I fix her breakfast, and although she used to protest vehemently, she now is happily content listening to the music, screeching when it suits her, and playing with a toy or two.

First, I found myself humming. By the next day, I was singing along with the tape. Now, by the time I exit the kitchen, I actually have a smile on my face. No kidding. I love "Wake up Toes." ("Wake up toes, wake up toes, wake up toes and wiggle, wiggle, wiggle.") Nevin is shocked at the change in me. The three of us now look like a bunch of loons singing and dancing around the house. I hope the neighbors can't hear. Then again, after all of that crying, it's probably a refreshing change.

Dad's Thoughts

The other day, Annie, Addie, and I went to a birthday party for Addie's cousin David. It was his third birthday and pretty typical of family gatherings of this sort—good food and plenty of it, half a dozen conversations going on at once, the kids screaming and running around (their parents often chasing them), and the grandparents sitting back and watching with amusement and the relaxed air of those who know it's someone else's turn to try to keep order.

Watching this circus, I couldn't help but recall similar gatherings when I was a child. The events were basically the same, although my perspective, of course, was radically different. Even the characters were about the same—never mind that the actors wore different faces.

The most entertaining to me was Lenny, perhaps because twenty years ago I played that role. He is the eldest son of Ann's sister, Sue. A tall, athletic, nine-year-old, Lenny is probably the quintessential boy: constantly active, predictably shy around adults, and the proprietor of a remarkable imagination—which occasionally gets him into trouble. Yet, despite his mental and physical meanderings, he is acutely aware of other children. He takes genuine interest in Adelyn and is very gentle with her. As the oldest of her cousins, I know he will have a big influence on her, and it is reassuring to know that he is both gentle and compassionate.

Since Adelyn's birth, I have become increasingly aware of the importance of family—extended family. Grandparents, aunts, uncles, and, especially, cousins can have a great effect on a child. The family provides a structural foundation, the tangible link to a child's history, and, ideally, reinforcement of basic values.

Cousins are contemporaries, playmates. If there is a significant difference in age (as with Lenny and Addie), cousins can be teachers—even role models. Aunts and uncles are often the first adults, other than parents, with whom the child develops relationships. Unhindered by the traditional child/parent roles, these relationships can sometimes develop into close, life-long friendships.

Grandparents, however, are in a class by themselves. They are the most important members of the extended family. Grandparents, besides being the only relatives legally permitted to spoil a child, provide a sense of history and a sense of identity because they know what the parent was like as a child. (And they remember with agonizing detail.) The stories your parents tell to your children fascinate them. I think it helps them further define who their parents are and bequeaths the link from their ancestors. Grandparents are a valuable resource, not only for children but for parents as well.

Addie is fortunate. We have a lot of family in the area and we see them often. With the Kishbaughs, it is only my immediate family—my brother and my father. Extended family get-togethers occur far too infrequently. Ann's fam-

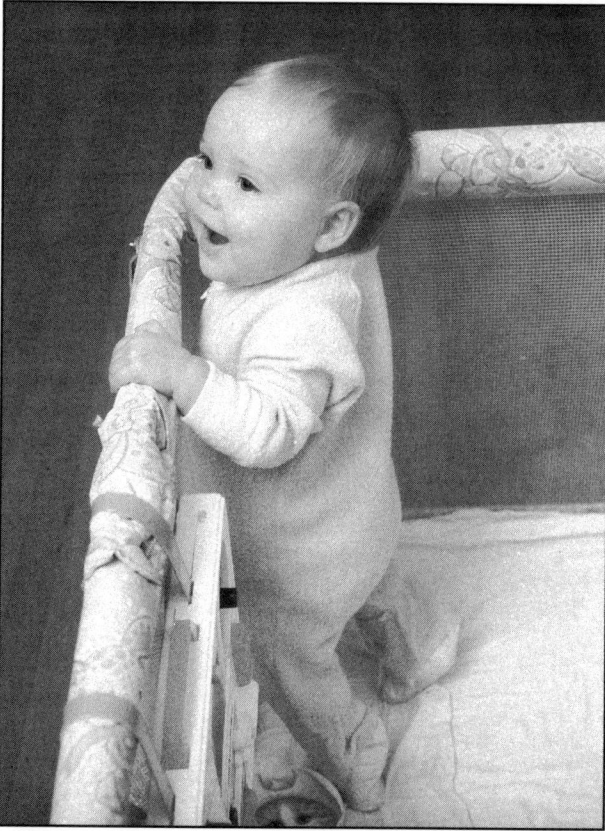

Singing along (sort of) to the music we play before breakfast.

ily, however, gets together six or seven times a year. I don't mean just immediate family, which would include Addie's aunts and uncles—the Sandt gatherings routinely include great-aunts and uncles, second cousins, and even one great-grandmother. These reunions are the result of Ann's grandfather's belief in the value of a close-knit family. The tradition is carried on by his sons and often includes as many as thirty people sitting down to dinner at once. The logistics, obviously, require some attention, but it's worth it. Besides, everybody pitches in. Family gatherings of this sort allow children to learn social skills in a comfortable setting. They also reinforce the basic values of cooperation and tolerance, not to mention the simple virtue of enjoying the company of family.

Family history, including the embarrassing anecdotes, is also important. Unfortunately, few of us recognize its value until after our children are born, if then. So many of the stories we heard as children from our parents, grandparents, aunts, and uncles get lost through our inattention. My mother knew all the details of our history, and I now regret not having listened more closely. Because of that, Adelyn will never hear some wonderful stories. But I plan to make sure that Adelyn has the chance to get to know her family—even distant relatives. My hope is that this will leave her with many fond memories, a sense of belonging, and an appreciation of her own history.

Eleventh Month—Pediatric Commentary by Dr. Marie Keith

The art of listening to baby talk requires a cultivated ear. Parents are very adept learners when told what sounds to decipher.

By the eleventh month, most babies will be very "gabby." They'll produce a variety of sounds that are the stepping stones for speech. They've been practicing the yells and squeals that produce the vowel sounds and learned to move their lips and tongues to make many of the consonant sounds. In hearing spoken language, babies have heard rhythm, cadence and inflection, which they imitate in their nonsensical babble.

The true beginning of speech comes when a meaning can be attached to their utterances. Some of the earliest sounds that bear meaning are those for the mother and father. A crying baby in distress will often emit the "m" sound repetitively as "mamamamama." When the mother comes to the baby's aid, she may say something like, "Okay, baby Mama is here." Both the baby and the mother hear the "mama" sound as they each vocalize it, and in a very gradual transition, the baby begins to know that when she forms this sound, her mother or "mama" appears. This may be the first awareness a baby has that a sound she makes evokes a certain response.

The sound "dada" is an early vocal emission and, depending on the baby's ability to produce the sound, often precedes mama. "Dada" is said in a random manner for many things, usually to express delight and joy. If the parents realize that this sound, which represents a multitude of things, is the foundation for the word "daddy" and repetitively say "dada" to the child to indicate the father, she will soon produce this sound to draw the attention of the father. And when she realizes that producing this sound provokes a very predictable response from those around her, a light seems to go on in her brain as her speech center is activated.

Most babies have certain "best" sounds they produce and usually their first true words are from among these sounds. The environment in which a baby spends her day-to-day existence also influences the first words she will say. For example, if a child is raised in a home with a pet such as a cat or dog, this pet may be the object of intense curiosity. And if her best consonant sound is a "c," she may try to say "cat," or "dog" if her best consonant sound is a "d." And imitating the sounds that the animal makes is also a source of endless fascination and excitement for the baby and parent.

The initial attempt at a word will have the simple essence of the word, that is, a major consonant and vowel sound. So cat may be heard as "ca" dog as "daw." In listening for these simple, essential sounds, a parent can then recognize the baby's intent and point to the object saying its name fully. The baby will be delighted. The best consonant sound may then be used to form other words. If, for example, a baby has produced the sound "hi," she may then quickly learn words such as "hot," "hat," and "head."

"Bottle" is usually an important word for babies and the "b" sound is often an easy one to make. Many babies will say "baba" to mean bottle. The essence of the word is clear and the repetition of the sound correlates with the cadence of the syllables.

Babies listen to spoken language for a long time before they begin to make sense of it. When it is apparent that a baby has begun to understand that a specific meaning is attached to her sounds, it is important for the mom and dad to begin to speak the single word names of objects to her. Babies love to point to objects or people and hear their names. This is how they begin to integrate the sounds of words that allow them to develop a vocabulary. The more complex aspects of speech come much later, but at this early stage, the simple noun-form names of objects begin to appear.

In a very gradual manner, a shift begins to occur in the baby's conceptualization of her world as she moves from a pre-verbal to a verbal understanding of her surroundings. We begin to get an inkling of her ability to understand concepts when generic words appear such as "this" and "that." Or perhaps she may apply her word for "dog" to mean all four-legged creatures.

It is at this early stage of language development that picture books begin to have relevance for the baby. She will take great pleasure in sitting and looking at pictures in a book and hearing the names of the objects that they depict. Well before she is able to speak the words, she may be able to understand them and point to the named object.

The development of receptive and expressive language is an exciting milestone for the baby and something that all parents eagerly await. Listen carefully. That first word will take you by surprise!

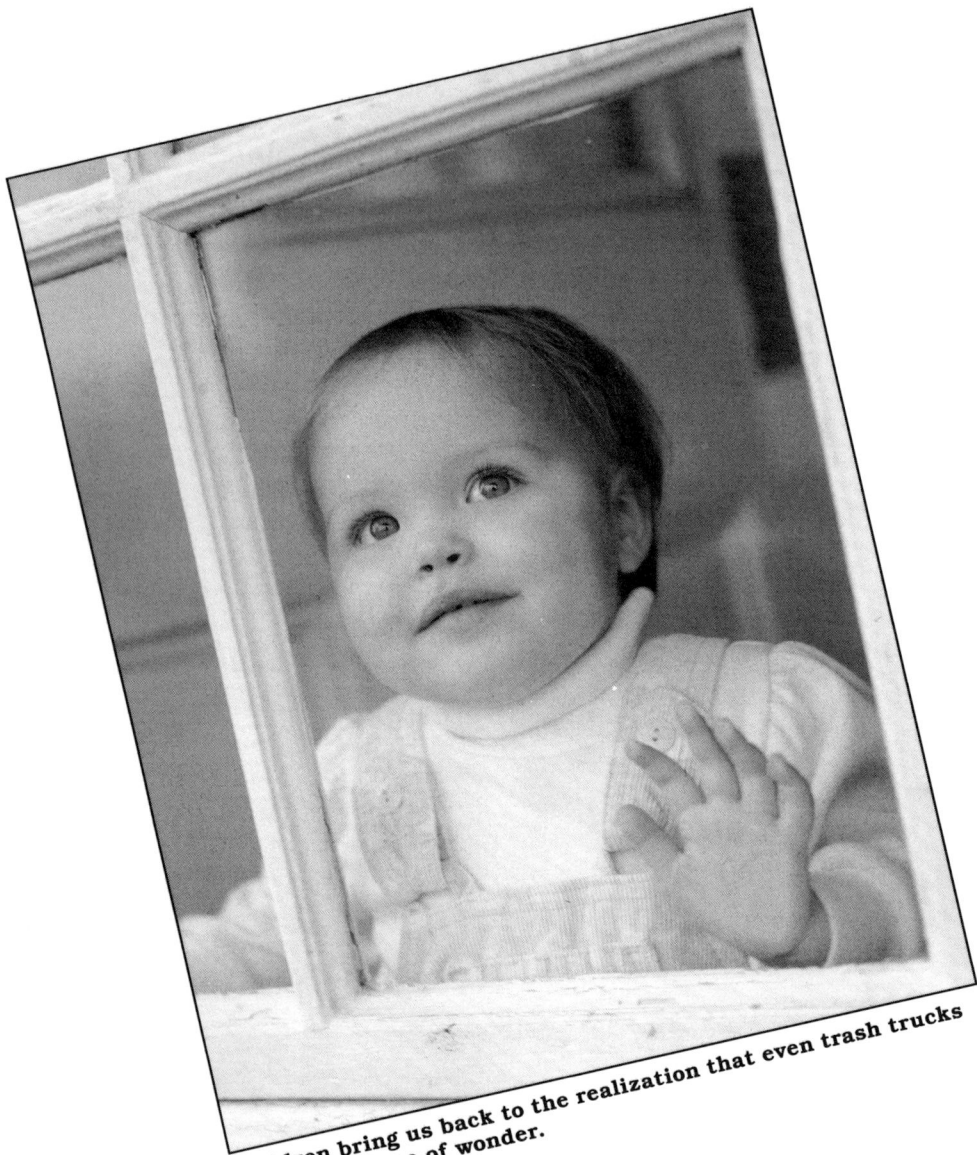

Children bring us back to the realization that even trash trucks can be a source of wonder.

Twelfth Month

Mom's Thoughts

"Nevin, baby needs a new pair of shoes." And with that said, we were off to the local shoe store as soon as our schedules would allow for Addie's first pair of shoes. She did not like them or the salesman who was trying to measure her particularly wide feet. Luckily, I was prepared with juice and a snack to divert her from the unpleasantries at hand. (I never leave home without a baby pretzel or two anymore.) While holding the wiggly Addie, I was amused to see another set of parents with their calm one-year-old who was taking the whole situation in stride. Once the shoes were on her feet, Addie seemed puzzled by them, but somewhat resigned. By the time Nevin had taken her over to the mirrors and play area in the shoe store, she was warming up to them. Addie is growing fonder of them with each passing day as she spends more and more time in a vertical position, and she has found that untying the laces is a big thrill. It keeps her amused during car trips very nicely.

Addie is standing a lot these days. She hasn't taken any steps forward yet, but she stands in midair balancing herself for long periods. She looks somewhat expectant and there is a gleam in her eye, but the courage to take that step is not fully developed yet. Encouragement from us makes her drop to her buns quickly, so we have learned to back off. She'll do it in her own time, thank you very much.

With her new sense of balance, she has become adept at helping me take her clothes off. When getting ready for her bath, she lifts her arms and legs appropriately to ease shirts and pants off while holding on to the tub with one arm. It's really cute. She always lifts her limbs in the same order. Right arm, left arm, right leg, left leg. "And, ready, off comes the diaper." Giggle, giggle. Addie also loves taking her clothes off in her crib—socks, pajama bottoms, loose pants.

One new skill this month that alleviates some of my worries is that Addie is able to back down the steps now. I still supervise her, but I now know that she can do it correctly. I have been showing her for some time now how to turn around and move her legs down from step to step, but she seemed disgruntled by my interference and continued to try to negotiate them head first. This had been going on for weeks, and I had just about given up on our lessons for the time being when she surprised me one day.

By mistake I had left the top stairway gate undone when we came upstairs to get her bath ready. Almost immediately after realizing what I had done, I ran in a panic to rectify the error. Just as I reached the gate, I saw Addie turning around on the top stair. I quickly took position on

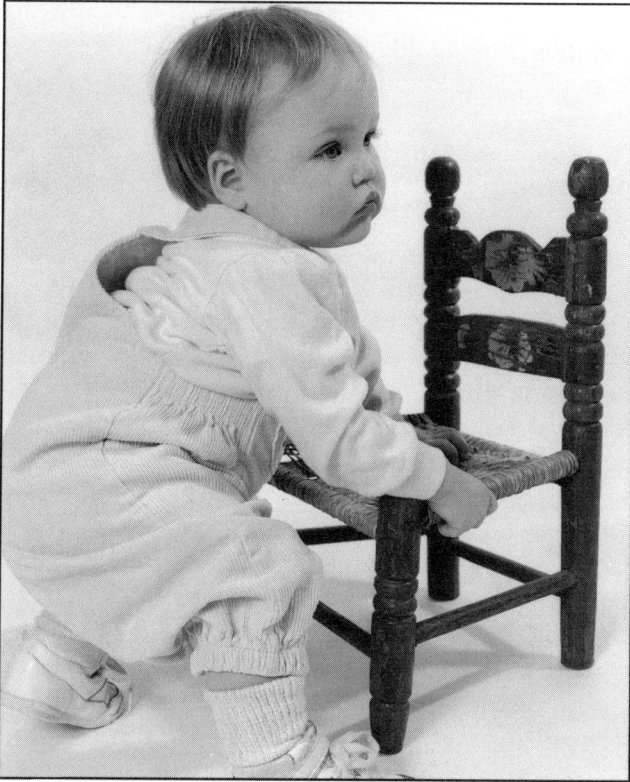

Adelyn's new shoes give her added support for standing and, soon, walking.

the stair below her. Sure enough, she did it exactly as I had shown her. Addie was really pleased with herself and is now delighted when she gets the chance to practice. She gets a big grin on her face when I invite her to come down the stairs. She has also made the connection on her own that it is a useful movement for coming down off of the couch or the bed. Pretty impressive, Addie.

This month Addie is obsessed with dragging things around with her—paper, toys, her clothes, our shoes—anything she can possibly lift. The bigger the better. She tries almost every object in the house, even taking each one up and down the staircase. She drops it, waves it, looks at it at odd angles, lets it fall a few steps, retrieves it, bangs it. Nothing is to mundane for her scrutiny.

When we go out on errands, she is like an octopus. I'll be talking with a clerk, and when I look down, Addie has grabbed something off the counter or is trying to sweep the counter of its contents. I have to keep the grocery cart in the middle of the aisle now and can't get too close to the shelves. You never know what may end up in the cart or in Addie's mouth. She also surprised me by standing up in the cart one day. I usually take one of my belts with me to the store to strap her in, although it hadn't really been necessary—until now. On this particular day, I knew it would only be a very quick trip so I left it in the car.

While talking with a friend I met, I looked over and there she was trying to leap over the back of the seat and into the cart. I quickly grabbed her. My heart missed a beat. I berated myself: strike two for Mom this month. I try to be so careful and keep abreast of the new skills she will be developing so I can anticipate situations. At times, however, I find myself accepting the status quo and taking it for granted. Luckily, there is a sort of mother's intuition. Mothers, parents really, can almost immediately sense danger in the air. We cannot, of course, rely on this solely, but thank God there is a back up for our humanness sometimes.

In the same way as accepting the status quo, as a mother it is hard to refrain from saying things such as "Addie doesn't like or like to do _____ ." I found myself saying this a lot in the beginning, probably as a way of getting to know her and feeling as if I knew her. But at this point, I can see that what Addie likes and what Addie can do changes almost daily. Addie couldn't stand in the cart yesterday, but she can today. Addie didn't like carrots yesterday, but she likes them today. Addie didn't want her morning nap yesterday, but she wants it today. I am constantly surprised by Addie. It's really hard to keep up with her. I guess I better just go with the flow (and watch her vigilantly).

One of Addie's favorite rituals is brushing her teeth. We started doing this when she developed enough teeth to warrant it, and she loves sucking and chewing on the toothbrush as I read her bedtime story. My dentist told me

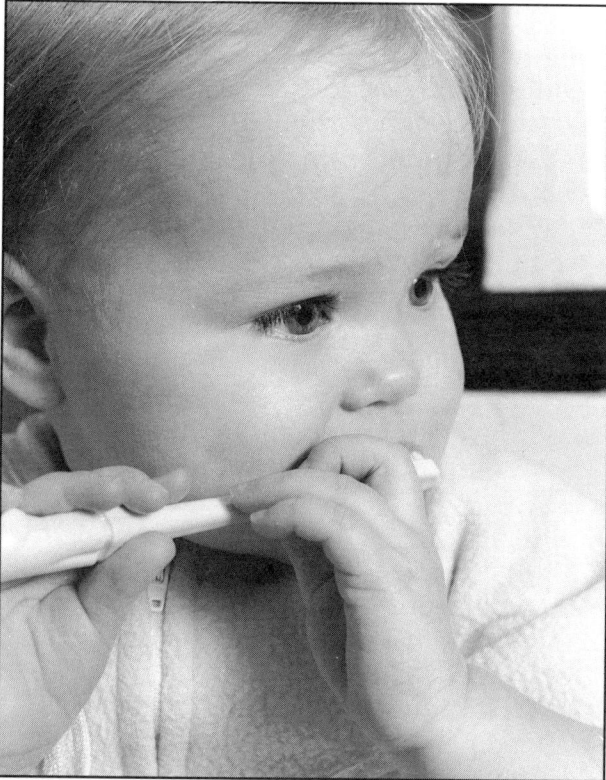

Part of her naptime and nighttime ritual is brushing her teeth. She doesn't brush so much as chew, but she is developing the habit.

recently that this activity isn't enough and that I need to get in there and really brush her teeth, then I can let her chew on the brush. This is not an easy task, but he stressed that it is better to get children used to this early because a parent needs to do this until the children are four or five years old at which time they finally develop the dexterity needed to handle the toothbrush correctly. We're making progress. Just recently, she opened her mouth and let me do it a few times without the customary struggle, but this could change tomorrow!

Addie also has been feeding herself with a spoon lately. We need to fill it up for her every time, but she really seems to be enjoying it. The amount of food she eats is amazing. She has been having a late growth curve (almost five pounds and three inches gained in these last three months!) and appears to be making up for lost time. She will eat all her dinner (a huge plateful of meat, vegetables, and fruit), eight ounces of formula, and then polish off a bagel if it is given to her. The doctor is really pleased with her gains, and at her twelve-month check-up he showed me the striking upward curve on her growth chart.

Addie has not really spoken her first word consistently, but she goes through phases of saying a particular word. "Da-dee" is her favorite word this month, and she will repeat it after you say it. She will go to Nevin if I ask her, "Where is Da-dee?," so I know she understands the word. She also understands a considerable number of commands: "Give to Mommy." "Come here, Addie." "Stand up, please." "Sit down." I find that I can talk to her about events that will happen, such as her bath, using key words like "splish-splash" and "rubber ducky," etc. I can tell she knows what I'm talking about by the grin on her face and the way she flails her arms and legs.

Adelyn is particularly intrigued with Richard Scary's picture books that are heavily laden with many characters and things. I actually wouldn't have thought that these books would be of interest to her because they are so busy, but she found one of my niece's old books on her bookshelf, and she is mesmerized. I frequently ask her to point out things on the page. Common items such as cats and dogs are usually found. She doesn't find the other things correctly, but I praise her just the same. Addie loves the game, and the interaction is reinforcing her already strong interest in books.

This is a fun age. Addie enjoys sharing. She learns more with each passing day. She plays well by herself. She listens when you tell her "No" (although I understand that this will change dramatically in the next few months—or possibly days). She truly enjoys other people (her separation anxiety has lessened considerably). And she shows affection at times. I got a kiss last week—the warmest little breath and softest little lips brushed my cheek ever so gently. In a way I wish I could keep her this age because I am having so much fun, but I know that there is a lot more fun to come. This is really only the beginning.

Dad's Thoughts

I came in the door one day to find my daughter sliding backwards down from the first landing of our staircase. Ann was sitting calmly at the bottom.

"Whoa," I said, rushing over with both hands outstretched to catch her.

"Relax," Ann laughed. "She does this all the time."

"She does?"

"This is the fifth time today."

"I haven't been around much lately, have I?"

It's true. When I'm busy, I miss a lot of what's happening at home. That is, I miss a lot of what's happening with Adelyn. These days, even if I'm gone only a day or two, Addie has changed considerably.

On those afternoons I'm able to watch Addie (and give Ann a break), Ann has to brief me on my daughter's current schedule—as though I were a rookie parent again.

"She'll only go down for an hour nap in the morning now," Ann instructs me, "give her some diluted juice when she wakes up. Afternoons? I don't know what she'll do. She should take a nap around two o'clock maybe three, if not read her some books to give her a chance to relax. Also it's Tuesday, let her watch the trucks."

"What trucks?" I ask.

"The trash trucks. She loves 'em."

"Really? Why?"

"Who knows. But she does. It's funny. She hoots and hollers at them from the upstairs window."

But on those occasions I'm with her in the afternoon (or morning, depending on our schedules), I really enjoy her company. I no longer feel as though I'm just babysitting, taking care of the basics. We spend a good portion of the time laughing and wrestling. I hand her different toys to see

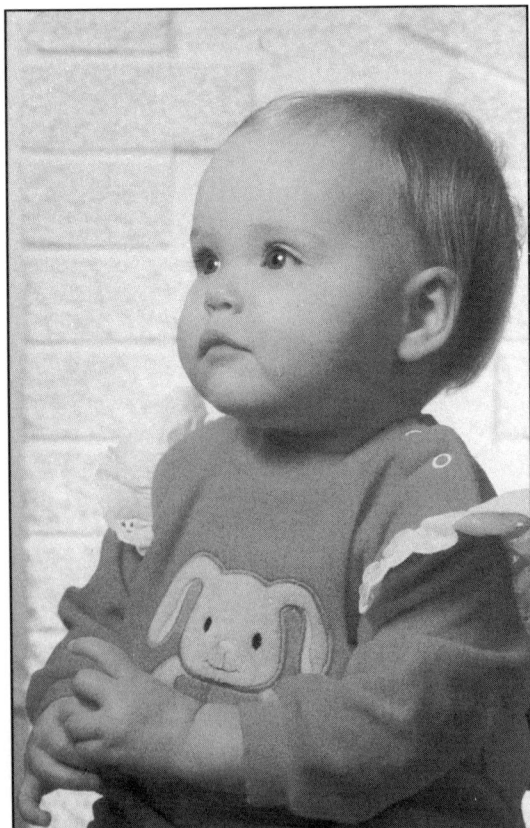

A portrait of Adelyn at one year.

how well she has learned to use them, or I'll crawl behind her pretending to chase her—I "tackle" her when I catch her and toss her into the air. She screeches and giggles; I laugh to see her laugh. Believe me, it beats working.

But, it is work. I don't know how many fathers get the chance to spend a whole day chasing after their kids, but by the end of the day, you will be exhausted. Play time is one thing, but add to that cleaning, feeding (which includes cooking), fighting to dress her, and running interference against table ends, pens, and other household dangers, and you have a very demanding job. Try reasoning with an irate one-year-old whose primary response to external stimuli is screaming. And we only have one. For those poeple who deal regularly with two, three, or four kids at a time, all day—well, they are true heroes as far as I'm concerned.

I suppose, as with anything else, the operation becomes somewhat streamlined with practice, but, at the end of the day, I still come away with great respect for Ann's patience and ability. (By the way, on top of all of the above, Ann also has to squeeze in a few hours on the computer during the day.)

If all this sounds like complaining, it's not. It's simply reality. Children can and will be maddening at times; children are a true test of your patience and endurance. But, and here's the payoff, they can, in an instant, make you forget about all the bad stuff. A glance, a laugh, or simply peeking in on them while they sleep will wipe away three hours of incessant screaming or let you ignore the oatmeal that found its way into your shoe. Their charm is natural, unpremeditated; there are no agendas here, no tactics. (We were all that way once.)

In the evening, before supper, the three of us gather in her "playroom," which is just off the kitchen. Ann and I just sit on the floor and watch her play while dinner is cooking. It gives us a chance to talk and be with her at the same time. Between activities, she crawls over to one of us, scrambles to a standing position to look us in the eye, grins and bounces on her toes. Then she drops to her rump and wanders toward some object that has suddenly caught her interest. She returns a few minutes later and dives into my lap with a giggle. I stop talking with Ann to turn Addie upside down or tickle her. It is very effective downtime. Regardless of the kind of day its been, twenty minutes of this and I feel great again.

For me, that is the true charm of children—they are rejuvenating. Through them, we see the world as new again. At the time in our lives when the monotony of daily living—of bills and taxes and too much work—has left us jaded, they come along and let us be kids again. They bring us back to the realization that even trash trucks can be a source of wonder.

Twelfth Month—Pediatric Commentary by Dr. Marie Keith

Our young family has come to the end of a year of many firsts. The true magic of the year has been seeing with adult eyes, and sharing with the baby, all the freshness and wonder of first-time achievements.

The first birthday will mark the end of an incredible year of initiation into parenthood and family life. It usually is a time for much reflection on the joys and happiness and the fears and anxieties that came with being new parents. Looking back, we see an enormous amount of growth and the achievement of many developmental milestones for baby and parents.

Physically, the baby is now a sturdy little person who has outgrown untold numbers of baby outfits. Developmentally, we have seen her learn to smile, use her hands, roll over, sit, crawl, cruise, hold her bottle, attempt to feed herself, babble, and perhaps say her first words. Socially, she has learned to laugh, vocalize with others, recognize familiar faces and show some shyness with strangers, and appear somewhat anxious when separated from the comforting arms of Mom and Dad. Reminiscing on all the accomplishments of the year, it sometimes seems that it was eons ago when the baby was a tiny newborn. Yet at other times it seems that she has grown up in the twinkling of an eye.

When we look at what parents accomplish in the first year, the list is no less astonishing. They grow from feeling nervous and insecure in handling their newborn to being confident and able in dealing with most of the daily issues of child care. They have mastered the routines of feeding, bathing, changing diapers, and dressing their baby. They have learned to soothe the baby's cries, help her with her sleeping problems, and comfort her through teething, minor illnesses, and those inevitable bumps and bruises that come with the adventure of movement.

By far the most significant growth for the parents was the adjustment of their adult lives to accommodate the needs of a growing baby and to form a family. They learned important lessons in sharing, giving, sacrificing, patience, and, when necessary, letting go. They learned the importance of finding time for each other and time for themselves. Growing through the first year of parenthood causes much evaluation of self and redefinition of adult roles. Coming through all these changes, parents are truly initiated into the institution of family life.

But as you probably can guess, this initiation is just the beginning. Although the first year had a myriad of wonderful events, it simply laid the foundation for the adventures to come. The years ahead will be no less exciting as the baby grows into a toddler, a preschool-age child, a school-age child, and, finally, a teenager. But in the same way that Ann and Nevin understood each stage as it arose, the lessons in the years to follow as they raise Addie will come in an orderly fashion.

The next stage that parents of a twelve-month-old can anticipate is her first steps in walking alone. By now she has been practicing cruising, walking while holding on to something or with someone holding her hands. Sometimes she may momentarily let go and be balanced enough to stand alone for a few seconds. The process toward walking takes some daring and many babies approach it very cautiously. At first, she may take one step from a secure place to another, perhaps going from the arms of Mom to the arms of Dad.

One of these days, when she's ready, she will go from taking one step to taking three or four steps and then soon, she'll be walking across a room. For a short time, crawling will continue to be her preferred mode of rapid movement as she gains confidence in her balance for walking. She will practice it more and more and earn her new name as a toddler. Happy Birthday, Addie! Happy Birthday, Ann and Nevin! It's been a great year.

Tenth through Twelfth Months— Child Development Commentary by Dr. Anita Hurtig

It seems amazing to parents that just as babies grow adept at moving away by crawling and walking, they also demonstrate strong signs of wanting to stay close. Ann calls this "separation anxiety." It is a normal, expected behavior at this point in development. This apparent paradox represents the pull between two systems: exploratory and attachment. Both are appropriate and essential for normal development but stir up for Addie disturbing conflict. How to move out, but stay safe. As Ann describes it, "when she is in uncertain territory, she looks for fortitude."

Separation anxiety arises out of at least two major developmental accomplishments. One is object permanence—a cognitive process that emerges as the baby is able to "hold on" to the image or memory of her mother, even in her absence. At this state, however, Addie doesn't understand that once gone, mother will also return. This awareness that mammas and other objects do return comes with object constancy, a recognition Addie will soon develop, which signals the diminution of separation anxiety in most normally developing children.

The second essential process for separation anxiety to be manifested is attachment. As we have seen all along in Addie's development, she is becoming increasingly "attached" to Ann and Nevin, signalled by her yearning to make contact, their capacity to regulate her moods, and, most of all, her affective responses (smiling, kissing, and even biting). Addie's difficulty in falling asleep without Ann and Nevin present is a common feature of separation anxiety. Falling asleep is a fearful separation experience for most babies, and they will often fight it by demanding that one parent or another protect them from this fear of the unknown—of the loss of their powerful protective presence. With time, as Addie recognizes that she does wake up— that she and mommy and daddy are "constant"—the fear becomes neutralized. Ann and Nevin have suffered the inevitable pain of waiting for their baby to build the cognitive and affective structures to cope with the deep and underlying anxiety which any loss—real or imagined—stirs up.

In sharing Ann and Nevin's experiences, we gain the sense that by Addie's first birthday much of their initial anxiety has been calmed, and they have a more realistic and relaxed approach to their baby. Ann's description of Addie's appetite is a wonderful metaphor for Addie's appetite for taking in every aspect of her surroundings. Her blossoming language development is the most dramatic evidence of the surge in cognitive development which is occurring now. The crucial element in this accomplishment is the interaction which Ann so imaginatively describes and tenderly nurtures —the constant dialogue between mother and child. Ann responds to Addie's cues, knowing that Addie knows and understands. Addie, in response, picks up Ann's cues: her pointing, her smiles, her words.

What Ann and Nevin recognize at some level is that getting through infancy with Addie is a constant test of all of their capacity to withstand frustration, failure, and fear. What makes it all possible is the ability to experience support and intimacy together. The result is what Erik Erikson has termed the accomplishment of the major task for the infant-parent triad in the first year of life—the development of trust. Addie has learned to do so much in this first year— to ambulate, to manipulate, to reach and to achieve, to communicate with gesture and expression and be understood. All of this culminates in her achieving a sense of reliability and predictability in the world around her, as represented by Nevin and Ann. It is this basic trust that ensures that Addie will be able to venture forth toward further evaluation and learning. Infants who have not experienced the constant, attentive, and respon-

sive care that Addie has, who are uncertain about the presence and attention of their parent(s), are less likely to move forward toward the major tasks of the second year of life—expanding their physical prowess, seeking out relationships with others, and communicating through language.

Ann and Nevin have discovered one of the most crucial aspects of parenting—the ability to gain assurance and comfort, as well as a sense of history, from one's own parents. Addie's grandparents are helping to fulfill some of Addie's needs that parents can't. They can be indulgent, comforting, and relaxed, offering a long-term perspective and accumulated wisdom. T. Berry Brazelton, a noted pediatrician and child developmentalist, has pointed out that each generation acts as a back-up for the next, helping young families to feel part of a culture with values and long-term goals. There are, however, natural hazards in the grandparenting process, which Addie's grandparents are clearly sensitive to, the fine line between involvement and intrusion. The key to balancing involvement and intrusion is conveying approval of baby *and* parents, joy in the child's accomplishments, and reliable but non-judgmental support of the parents.

Ann and Nevin are in for an exciting time. Erikson describes the baby's major task of the next twelve months as gaining a sense of autonomy—that is, of independence and closeness, of self-expression and awareness of others. Addie will be increasingly able to tell Ann and Nevin what she needs and how she feels. They've had to do much mutual guessing over these first twelve months, but as Nevin so perceptively states " . . . our child is not quite as fragile as we thought the first time we held her. We know that mistakes will be made . . . but they probably won't be fatal." Children are incredibly resilient, but parental sensitivity and constancy are vital. After sharing these exciting months with Addie, Ann, and Nevin, I feel confident in sharing Nevin's simple conclusion, "Addie *is* fortunate."

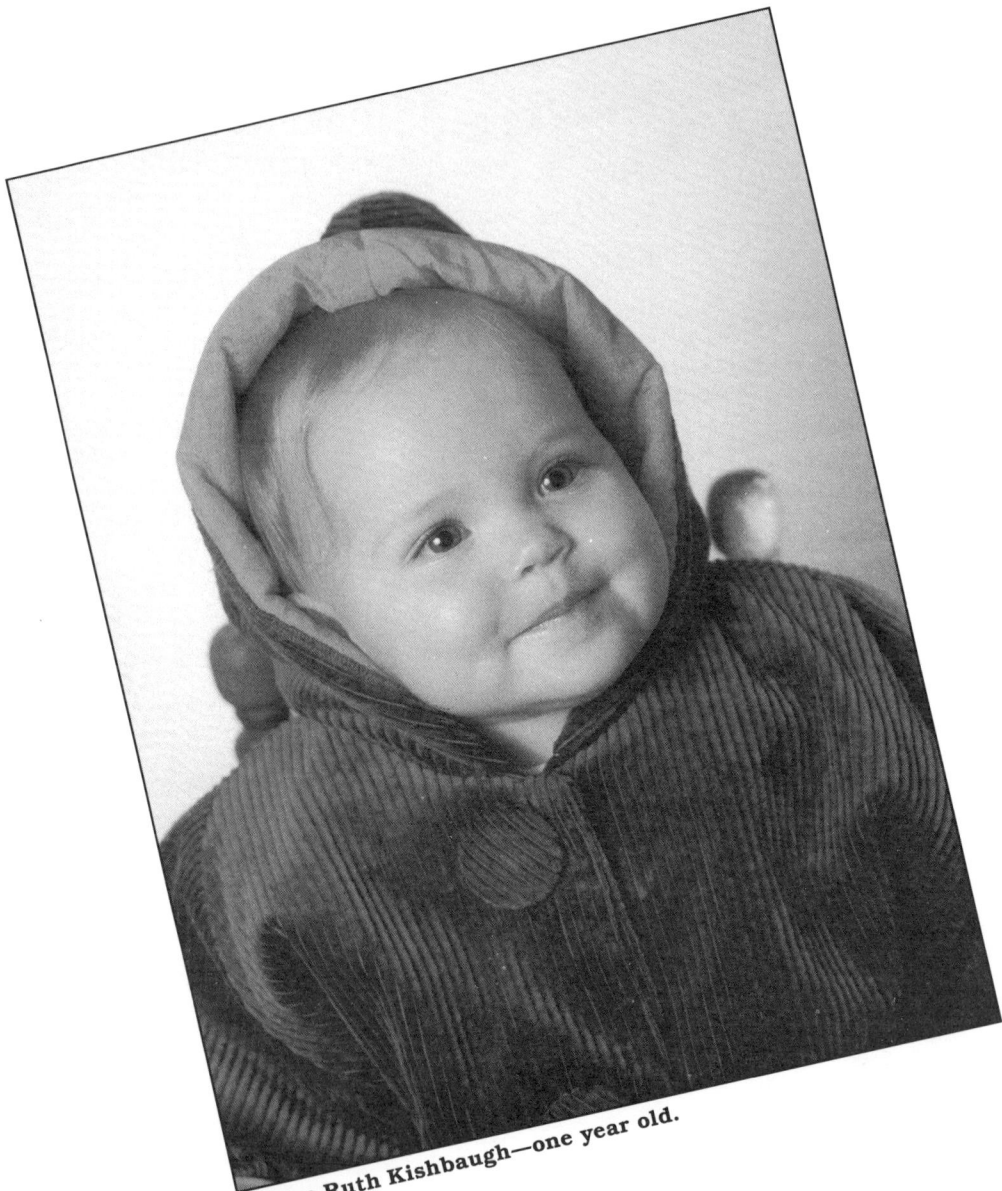

Adelyn Ruth Kishbaugh—one year old.

Happy Birthday

Mom's Thoughts

Well, here we are—fourteen
pounds and ten ounces, eleven
inches, eight teeth, and one emerging personality later. Adelyn
Ruth is becoming quite a character, and as Nevin so aptly said recently, "Addie gets the joke now."
She laughs readily and with
such infectious childlike glee. All
of this is such a change from
that wee infant we held in our
arms one year ago. (And my
arms can attest that twenty
pounds and twenty-nine inches

is a big change from five pounds, six ounces and eighteen inches.)

Looking back, I can see that with each accomplishment she made this past year, her spirit grew tenfold. While in some ways, we are wistful for that tiny little baby who just wanted to be cuddled and who smelled so wonderfully of sweet milk, in other ways we can't wait to see what the future holds for his little person perched on the edge of toddlerhood.

As for me, I am truly a mother now. I remember my father-in-law telling Nevin and me not long after we had Adelyn that having a baby is like falling in love all over

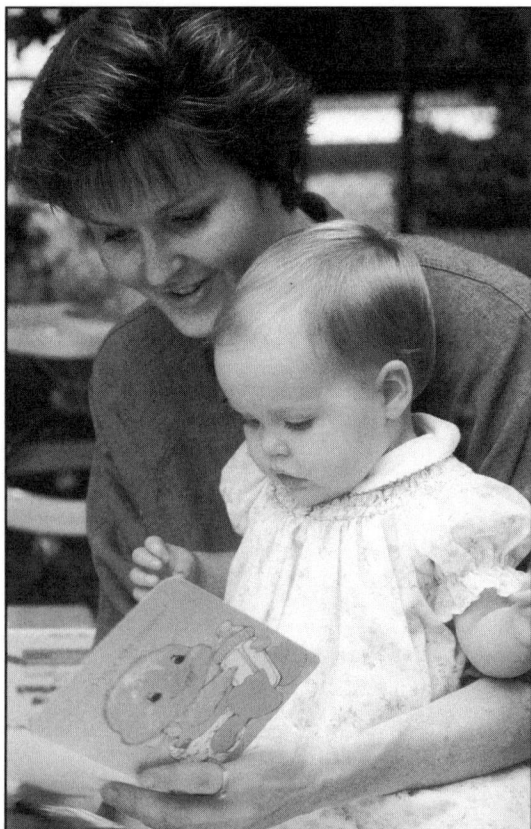

Annie and Addie reading one of her birthday cards.

again. I nodded my head and gazed adoringly at our child. However, from the perspective of a year past, I can see the similarities very clearly now. At the beginning, you are on cloud nine. (In fact, we were probably pretty sickening to a lot of people.) "Isn't she the most beautiful thing you ever saw." "I'm just crazy about her." "She is so good." There is no reality. It is only you and your wonderful husband with this adorable infant. You talk like an easy-listening radio station. (Don't you just remember being like that when you fell in love with your husband?) I can still recall that both of these beginnings produced the most wonderful feelings in the world. It must be what runner's talk about when they try to describe a "runner's high." For mothers especially, the birth of a child is the culmination of a nine-month-long marathon.

A few weeks go by and then some hints of reality break through the happy scenario. The baby is not perfect. The baby cries incessantly at times. The baby takes up so much time that there is no time for anyone else. I remember weeping to Nevin, "I really love being able to take care of her, but I don't get to spend any time with you anymore." You still love your baby dearly, but perhaps more clearly. It is about this time that you start speaking to friends in this manner: "I love her (him) dearly but there are times when I get so frustrated because _____ (fill in the blank)." You feel as if your complaining about any aspect of your baby or your care for her is like treason, so you qualify everything with "I love her dearly but. . . ."

Then you begin to notice that other people also discuss their children in less-than-glowing terms, but they clearly love their children and want the best for them. It is okay to put one's feet back on the ground and begin to really take on the role of mother and father. As Nevin's mother once said to a very young and a very bad Nevin: "I'll always love you but I won't always love what you do."

No, I'm not humming "Feelings" anymore, but I am mellower. Being awed by the miracle of life does change your outlook on the world for all time. Hearing "Pomp and Circumstance" the other day on the radio brought a mist to my eyes that would not have been there two years ago. It's funny, but every day after the birth you grow apart. Luckily, it is a very slow process encompassing eighteen or so years; but when I think back on how dependent she was on us for every factor of her life and how even now she can do many things on her own, it makes me both proud and a tiny bit misty. Yes, I'm a mother now.

Maternal Grandparents Thoughts

Watching our girls raise their children, we are struck by the differences in attitudes from when we were young parents. Like young parents everywhere at that time, we went by the book (Dr. Spock) or followed our family pattern and copied what our parents had done to us and our siblings. We admire and delight in watching the emotional involvement and love displayed by both parents now. As a young father, I didn't have time to see or enjoy my girls being raised. I usually worked two or three jobs and was using my GI bill to go to school at night. (My father had done the same during the Great Depression.) Also, it just wasn't the fashion for the father to be that involved in his child's rearing.

In addition, the thinking of the time seemed to reduce the process to more of a mechanical one instead of an emotional one. For example, if you cried, we followed this recipe: a) was it gas? we patted and burped you; b) diaper need changing? c) was a pin sticking you from the diaper? d) was there a temperature indicating an illness? If none of the above, we simply let you cry. The thought was that a person could spoil a baby with too much picking up.

Well, all of our girls survived thanks to their mother's good nurturing instincts, and we managed to raise three fine daughters, but what a shame that it could not have been different. We are so delighted to see the sharing of love and emotional support in our daughters' families. Perhaps

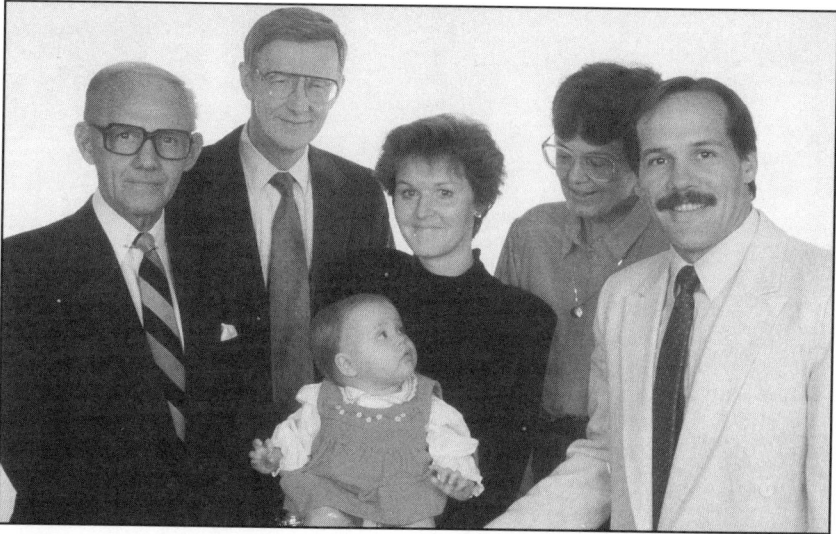

A family portrait on Addie's birthday. From left, Jack Kishbaugh, Lloyd Sandt (Ann's father), Annie, Liz Sandt, me, and, of course, Adelyn.

our example did teach them something very important: Take what we have given you and improve on it. Keep up the good work, girls (and, especially, you boys).

Paternal Grandfather's Thoughts

Like everyone, I had heard all the great things about being a "Grandparent." Of course, it was intriguing to me to contemplate an offspring of my own children—seeing in the second generation characteristics of my wife and me, and, of course, seeing the way my children would handle the many joys and problems of raising their own children. I used to tease them and say that when I saw them coming over for a visit with their "noisy, sticky-fingered" little ones I would lock the door and pretend not to be home.

When my daughter-in-law (Ann) became pregnant and my wife (Ruth) and I realized we would soon have a grand-

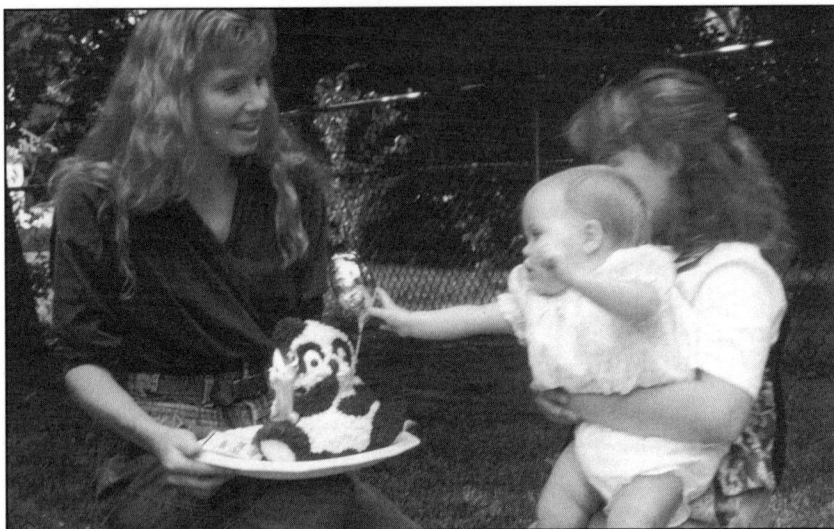

Aunt Sue brings Addie her first birthday cake. Of course, the balloon is what caught her attention.

child, it took on a new and wonderful meaning. Ruth at the time was suffering from cancer and her life, as you might expect, was far from pleasant. Her bedridden days of pain and general malaise were brightened by the prospect of this new child in the world. My own good feelings about my grandchild were enhanced because I saw the wonderful effect it had on Ruth.

Unfortunately, Ruth passed away eleven days before the baby was born. Ann and Nevin thoughtfully named the baby after her. My wife's name was Ruth Adelyn. Adelyn Ruth almost immediately came to be called "Addie," which was a nickname my wife always loved. I know I subconsciously look at Addie hoping to see things that are like her Grandmother Ruth, and I really do see some physical resemblances. Perhaps as she grows older, we will see similar personality traits as well.

Although the pain of my wife's death is still very strong, the presence of my granddaughter has helped me through this difficult time. Nevin and Ann live nearby and are most generous in visiting me. I see the baby frequently, and the time I spend with her is quite valuable to me. Watching the baby grow, having her respond to me, and seeing the joys she brings Nevin and Ann are truly the great rewards of being a grandfather. All the great things I've heard about having a grandchild are true. I only hope I can make a favorable contribution to her life. And though Addie will never know her grandmother, I know that somehow Ruth's influence will be felt.

For the moment I am thankful that God has allowed Addie to be a happy, healthy child with loving and caring parents and for the time I can spend with her.

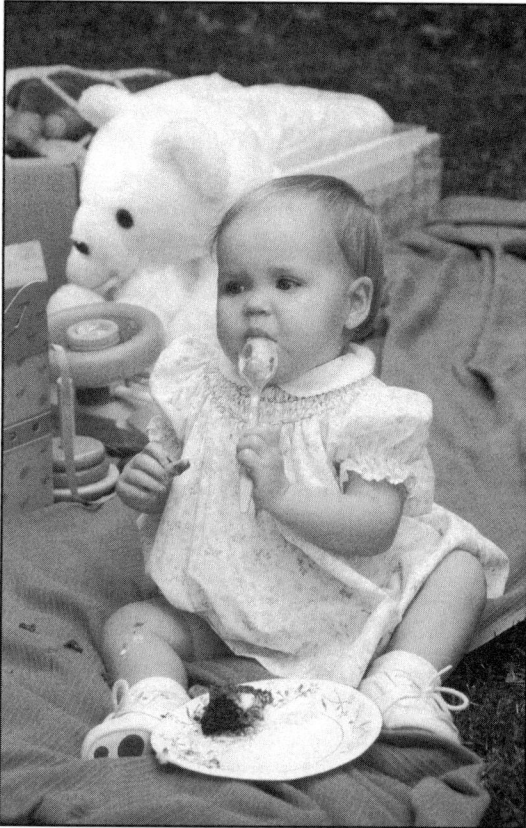

Presents stacked behind her, Addie tries a spoonful of cake.

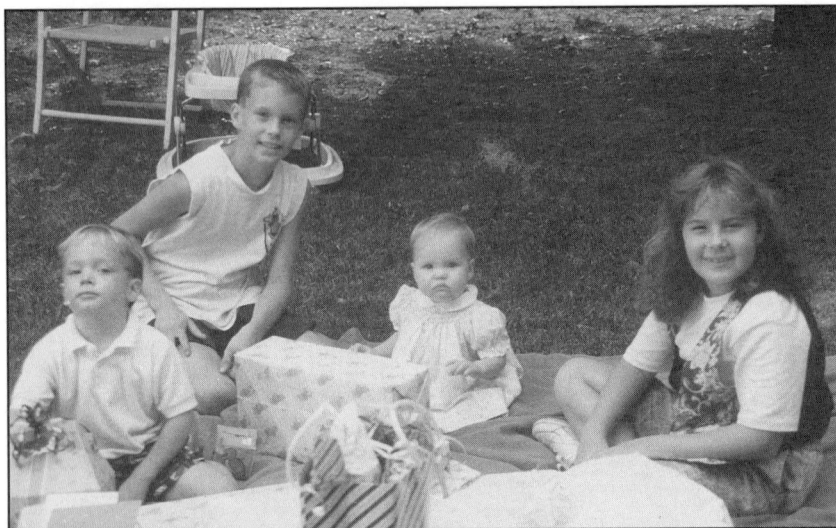

Adelyn and her cousins. From left, David, age three, Lenny, nine, Addie; and Amy Ruth, eight. They *love* birthdays.

Dad's Thoughts

Well, Adelyn is a year old. Of course, we had a party for her. Aunts, uncles, cousins, and grandparents all gathered for the occasion. But to tell the truth, Addie, the guest of honor, couldn't have cared less. In fact, she seemed a little put out by all the fuss. But these occasions are more for the parents and grandparents than for the little one.

The arrival of the first birthday is a great milestone—for the Mom and Dad as much as for the baby. It means they are no longer rookies; they have survived to become veteran parents. They can now discourse with authority on the subjects of diapers, teething, and Dr. Spock—not to mention the more advanced parenting courses, such as sleep deprivation and separation anxiety. This transition does not make us more interesting (people at cocktail parties still consciously avoid us), but it does make us more realistic.

We realize now that our child is not quite as fragile as we thought the first time we held her. We know that mistakes will be made, however hard we try to avoid them, but they probably won't be fatal. We understand that when a child ignores her parents, it's only because she is busy learning something else (although this doesn't apply to teenagers: when they are ignoring you, they are really ignoring you).

All kidding aside, the first birthday really is important. We can relax a bit now, our child has begun to be a person. We have started her on her way, but just as with a child riding a bike for the first time without training wheels, we'll have to run along side for while, just to be sure.

It's hard for me to remember now how tiny she was when I first held her, how helpless she was those first few months. Reviewing these chapters, seeing the pictures, really helps relive those moments. I think the benefits of having to analyze and articulate our thoughts over the past twelve months will accrue over the years. Annie and I will come back to these pages as the years go by and be very grateful to have our thoughts on paper. At the outset, we thought that it would be Adelyn who would derive the greatest benefit, but I see now that we have really done this for ourselves.

Index

US Bank
2010
$471.⁴³
Interest